IoT, Blockchain, and Smart Healthcare

The book examines the integration of Internet of Things (IoT), blockchain, and smart healthcare, providing a comprehensive analysis of these advanced technologies and their impact on the healthcare industry. It offers practical examples of how blockchain and IoT devices can be used to address real-world healthcare challenges and overcome the hurdles of implementing them in the healthcare sector.

IoT, Blockchain, and Smart Healthcare: Integration Techniques and Case Studies provides a detailed exploration of how these technologies are combined, giving readers a deep understanding of their role in revolutionizing healthcare. It explores the practical applications of blockchain and IoT devices in solving healthcare problems and addresses the challenges of incorporating these technologies into healthcare systems. The book also provides practical guidance on implementing cutting-edge methodologies, enabling readers to apply theoretical knowledge in real-world situations effectively.

By bridging the gap between technology and healthcare, this book makes complex concepts understandable to a wide audience, including healthcare professionals, researchers, technology enthusiasts, and policymakers.

Innovations in Health Informatics and Healthcare: Using Artificial Intelligence and Smart Computing

Series Editors: Rashmi Agrawal, Manav Rachna International Institute of Research and Studies, and Mamta Mittal, G.B. Pant Government Engineering College

The aim of this series is to publish reference books and handbooks that will provide conceptual and advanced reference material centered around Health Informatics and Healthcare using AI and Smart Computing. There are numerous fields within the healthcare sector where these technologies are applicable including successful ways of handling patients during a pandemic time. Large volumes of data, data analysis, smart computing devices like IoT for sensing health data have drastically changed the way the healthcare sector functions. The scope of the book series is to report the latest advances and developments in the field of Health Informatics with the use of the latest technologies. Each book will describe in detail the use of AI, Smart Computing, Evolutionary Computing, Deep Learning, and Data Analysis in the field of Health Informatics and the books will include real-life problems that focus on the Healthcare System.

Intelligent Computing Applications for COVID-19
Predictions, Diagnosis, and Prevention
Edited by Tanzila Saba and Amjad Rehman

Blockchain for Healthcare Systems
Challenges, Privacy, and Securing of Data
Edited by Shiekh Mohammad Idrees, Paural Agarwal, and M. Afshar Alam

Healthcare Systems and Health Informatics
Using Internet of Things
Edited by Pawan Singh Mehra, Lalit Mohan Goyal, Arvind Dagur, and Anshu Kumar Dwivedi

Ambient Assisted Living (AAL) Technologies:
Transitioning from Healthcare 4.0 to Healthcare 5.0
Edited by: Rashmi Gupta, Xiomara Patricia Blanco Valencia, Lalit Mohan Goyal, and Jeetendra Kumar

IoT, Blockchain, and Smart Healthcare
Integration Techniques and Case Studies
Edited by Manoj Kumar, Urmila Pilania, Rohit Tanwar, Neelu Jyothi Ahuja, and Mazdak Zamani

For more information on this series, please visit: https://www.routledge.com/Innovations-in-Health-Informatics-and-Healthcare-Using-Artificial-Intelligence-and-Smart-Computing/book-series/CRCIHIHUAISM

IoT, Blockchain, and Smart Healthcare

Integration Techniques and Case Studies

Edited by

Manoj Kumar, Urmila Pilania, Rohit Tanwar,
Neelu Jyothi Ahuja, and Mazdak Zamani

CRC Press
Taylor & Francis Group
Boca Raton London New York

CRC Press is an imprint of the
Taylor & Francis Group, an **informa** business

Designed cover image: Shutterstock

First edition published 2026
by CRC Press
2385 NW Executive Center Drive, Suite 320, Boca Raton FL 33431

and by CRC Press
4 Park Square, Milton Park, Abingdon, Oxon, OX14 4RN

CRC Press is an imprint of Taylor & Francis Group, LLC

ISBN: 978-1-032-84002-4 (hbk)
ISBN: 978-1-032-84043-7 (pbk)
ISBN: 978-1-003-51093-2 (ebk)

DOI: 10.1201/9781003510932

Typeset in Times
by KnowledgeWorks Global Ltd.

Contents

Preface

The fast progress of technology has paved the way for revolutionary innovations that are redefining the future of healthcare system. At the heart of this transformation lies the convergence of artificial intelligence, Internet of Things (IoT), blockchain, and smart healthcare solutions. Together, these technologies offer unmatched opportunities to enhance patient care, optimize healthcare system, and ensure data security. *IoT, Blockchain, and Smart Healthcare* researches into the complex relationship between these emerging fields, highlighting their applications, benefits, and challenges in modern healthcare. IoT has transformed healthcare system by enabling real-time monitoring, remote patient care, and predictive analytics. Smart medical devices, wearable technology, and connected sensors are transforming how diseases are diagnosed and cured, allowing for a more adapted approach to patient care. However, with this increased connectivity comes the pressing need for robust data security and integrity – an area where blockchain technology plays a critical role. Blockchain, with its decentralized architecture, offers a game-changing solution for securing healthcare data, improving interoperability, and ensuring transparency in medical records. By integrating blockchain with IoT, healthcare systems can alleviate cybersecurity risks, strengthen patient privacy, and build greater trust among all the stakeholders.

This book provides a comprehensive study of the synergy between artificial intelligence, IoT, blockchain, and smart healthcare. It covers fundamental concepts, real-world case studies, emerging trends, and key challenges that must be addressed to unlock the full potential of these technologies. Whether you are a researcher, practitioner, policymaker, or technology enthusiast, this book equips you with valuable insights and practical knowledge to navigate this rapidly evolving landscape. As healthcare stands on the crossover of a technological revolution, understanding and leveraging these innovations are crucial to improving patient outcomes and building a more efficient, secure, and accessible healthcare system. We hope this book serves as a guiding resource in your journey to implementing IoT and blockchain-driven smart healthcare solutions. We extend our heartfelt appreciation to the contributors whose knowledge, expertise, and passion have enhanced this book, as well as to the readers who broaden this scholarly journey with us.

Contributors

Ambika Aggarwal
University of Petroleum and Energy Studies
Dehradun, India

Shakeel Ahamad
NIET, Greater Noida
UP, India

Mamta Arora
Manav Rachna University
Faridabad, India

Satya Prakash Awasthi
Amity University
Gwalior, India

Ashutosh Bhatt
Swami Rama Himalayan University
Dehradun, India

Sovers Singh Bhist
NIET, Greater Noida
UP, India

R. Girija
MRIIRS
Faridabad, India

Shyam Bihari Goyal
City University Malaysia
Selangor, Malaysia

Ratneshwer Gupta
Software Quality Assurance Labs
Jawaharlal Nehru University
New Delhi, India

Shilpi Gupta
MRIIRS
Faridabad, India

Garima Jain
NIET, Greater Noida
UP, India

Prerna Kandpal
Manav Rachna University
Faridabad, India

Sumit Kumar Kapoor
Poornima University
Jaipur, India

Amanjot Kaur
Cardiff University
Cardiff, UK

Ajay Khunteta
Faculty of Computer Science
Poornima University
Jaipur, India

Aniket Kumar
MRIIRS
Faridabad, India

Manish Kumar
MRIIRS
Faridabad, India

Manoj Kumar
Manav Rachna University
Faridabad, India

Mrinal Pandey
Manav Rachna University
Faridabad, India

Urmila Pilania
Manav Rachna University
Faridabad, India

Deeya Rajput
School of Computer Science
University of Petroleum and Energy Studies
Dehradun, India

Dhruv Sharma
School of Computer Science
University of Petroleum and Energy Studies
Dehradun, India

Shikha Sharma
Department of Computer Science
Poornima University
Jaipur, India

Vijay Prakash Sharma
Manipal University
Jaipur, India

Sanjay Singh
Manav Rachna University
Faridabad, India

Shefali Singhal
MRIIRS
Faridabad, India

Rohit Tanwar
SMVDU, Katra
J&K, India

Deepak Uprety
NIET, Greater Noida
UP, India

Mazdak Zamani
State University of New York - Empire State University,
New York, USA

About the Editors

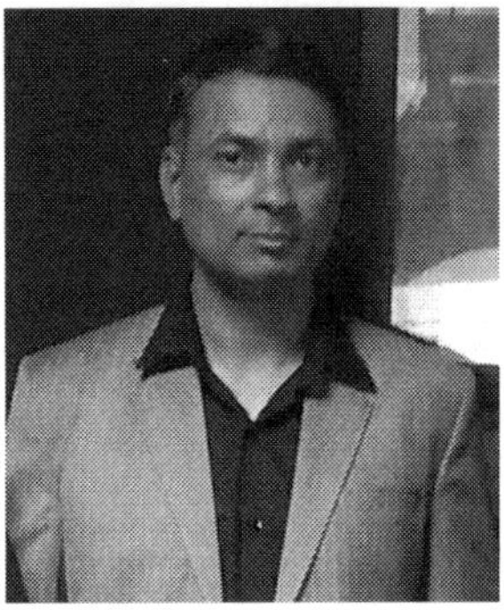

Manoj Kumar is presently working as Associate Professor in the Department of Computer Science and Technology, at Manav Rachna University, Faridabad. He has over 14 years of experience, including academics, industry, and research. He earned his PhD in 2022, in the area of Computer Vision. Dr. Kumar has published many research papers related to moving object detection and tracking in videos and also extracts features of moving objects/vehicles from video in real-time video surveillance systems. He has published more than ten papers in journals and has presented more than 40 papers at various international conferences. He has published four national patents, has participated in various workshops and faculty development programs, and has conducted various special sessions at many reputed conferences and workshops. His areas of expertise are Computer Vision, Artificial Intelligence, Machine Learning, Image Processing, IoT, and Blockchain.

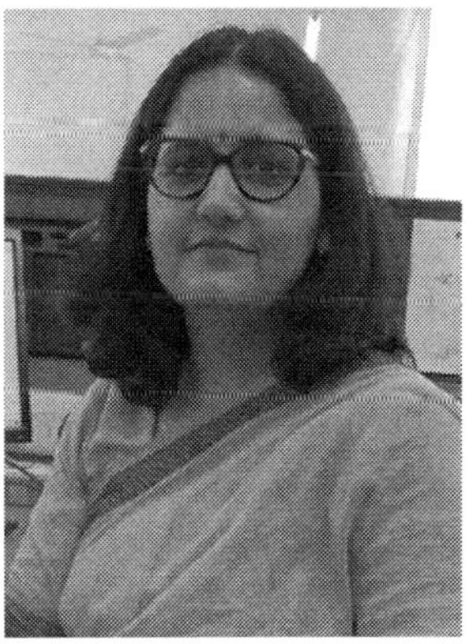

Urmila Pilania is currently working as Associate Professor in the Department of Computer Science and Technology, at Manav Rachna University, Faridabad. She has 14 years of experience in academics and research and received her engineering degree (B.Tech. in Computer Science and Engineering) in 2007 from Guru Jambheshwar University of Science and Technology, Hisar – Haryana (India). Dr. Pilania earned a master's degree (M.Tech. in Computer Science and Technology) in 2009 from Vaish College of Engineering, Rohtak – Haryana. She was awarded the doctoral degree (Ph.D. in Computer Science and Technology) in 2021 from Manav Rachna University, Faridabad, India. Dr. Pilania has published many research papers related to Information Security, object detection, and classification. She is the author of more than 46 research publications with journals/conferences of repute, and some papers are under review or in press for publication with leading publishers. She has published three national patents, three design patents, and three more are under examination. She has participated in various workshops and Faculty Development Programs and has also been associated with many conferences and journals as a reviewer and a member of their technical committee along with delivering guest lectures. Her primary research interests are in Information Security, Image Processing, Machine Learning, and Artificial Intelligence.

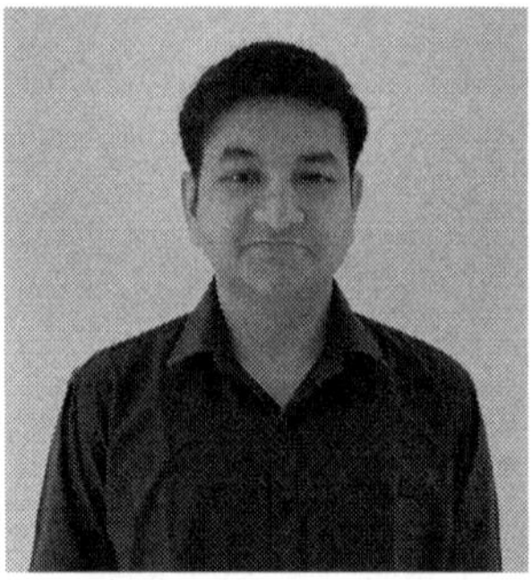

Rohit Tanwar received his bachelor's degree in Computer Science & Engineering from Kurukshetra University, Kurukshetra, India, and a master's degree in CSE from YMCA University of Science and Technology, Faridabad, India. He received his PhD in CSE from Kurukshetra University, Kurukshetra, and has more than ten years of experience in teaching. Currently, he is working as Associate Professor in the School of Computer Science and Engineering at Shri Mata Vaishno Devi University, Katra, J & K. He has more than 40 publications to his credit in different reputed journals and conferences, and his areas of interest include Network Security, Optimization Techniques, Human Computing, Soft Computing, Cloud Computing, and Data Mining.

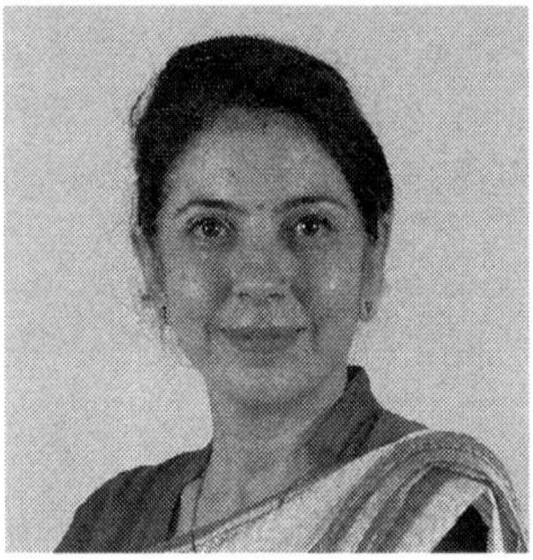

Neelu Jyothi Ahuja is Professor in the Department of Systemics, at the School of Computer Science at the University of Petroleum and Energy Studies, Dehradun. Her PhD was awarded in 2010, and apart from academic teaching at the university level (both at post-graduate and undergraduate levels), she is an active researcher. From the period of 2010–2017, she was head of the Research Centre-Computing Research Institute, spearheading intra-disciplinary research and coordinating research activities. To her credit, she has successfully delivered half a dozen R&D projects and consultancies funded by the Department of Science and Technology (DST), Government of India. She has been an invited speaker on various technical and research-oriented topics at widely acclaimed forums, both national and international, and is on the panel of various committees, including the World Health Organization -Promotion of Assistive Products and Technologies, and the DST-Expert Committee for Inspection and On-the-Spot Review of CORE (long-term) projects. She has also been a chair at various conference sessions and different internal and external meetings/forums. She holds 22+ years of experience in teaching, research, and project proposal development and has published papers in journals and conferences at international and national levels. Her areas of interest include Machine Learning, Intelligent Systems, Intelligent Tutoring Systems, Expert Systems, Artificial Intelligence, ICT, Object-Oriented Development, and Programming Languages.

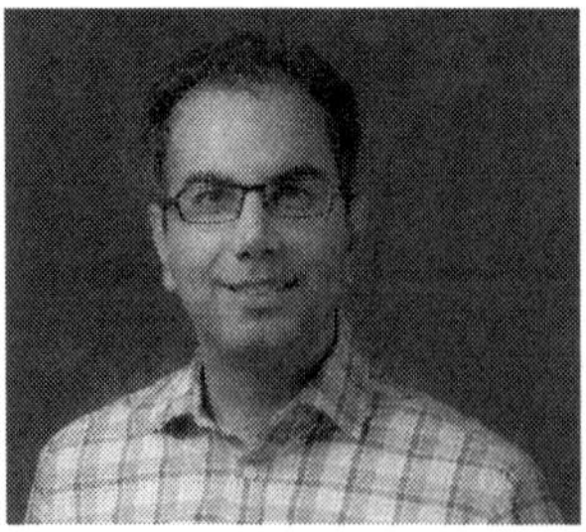

Dr. Mazdak Zamani earned his Ph.D. in Computer Science from Universiti Teknologi Malaysia (UTM) in 2011. He began his academic career as a Senior Lecturer at UTM's Advanced Informatics School, serving from 2011 to 2015. In 2015, he joined Wenzhou-Kean University as a full-time Assistant Professor in the Department of Computer Science. In Fall 2017, Dr. Zamani transitioned to Felician

University, where he served as an Assistant Professor of Cybersecurity and Computer Science. His exceptional contributions led to his promotion to Associate Professor of Cybersecurity in 2020. Since 2021, he has also been an Adjunct Professor at the Graduate Division of the Courant Institute of Mathematical Sciences at New York University, teaching graduate-level courses in Applied Cryptography and Network Security. In Fall 2024, Dr. Zamani joined Empire State University, part of the State University of New York system, as an Assistant Professor in the Department of Computer Science and Technology.

1 Introduction of IoT-Blockchain in Smart Healthcare

Manoj Kumar, Shyam Bihari Goyal, and Urmila Pilania

1.1 INTRODUCTION

In traditional healthcare management systems, registration of patients, billing of consultancy of doctors, prescriptions, record keeping, etc. are labor-intensive and require more time to complete the tasks. Hospital resources such as beds, staff, and equipment management are difficult by using traditional methods, resulting in delay and high cost. Patients are not able to access the online data because of traditional methods. The schedule of appointments with doctors for consultation, waiting time for consultation, and traveling to the hospital can be unconventional and time-consuming [1]. In the traditional healthcare system, the patient has to visit a doctor in the hospital for any type of consultation.

Health data of patients has to be collected manually when patients visit doctors, so continuous monitoring of patients is very rare. The continuous monitoring of patients utilizing Internet of Things (IoT) devices helps in the early identification of the disease. All types of care are provided in the hospital only when the patient visits the hospital physically. All the data of patients is stored in some centralized dataset, resulting in misunderstanding among doctors. The centralized data of patients without applying any modern data safety techniques may result in cyber-attacks. Data sharing among different systems or doctors may lead to imperfect patient histories.

IoT wearable devices are utilized these days for the collection of patient's activity levels, sleep patterns, and health data, which provide a comprehensive view of patient health. Due to the use of advanced techniques, remote monitoring of patients is very easy, resulting in reduced visits to hospitals. Blockchain confirms the security of a patient's data and stores the records in a decentralized manner. Blockchain's unchallengeable ledger avoids illegal access to patient data. Continued patient monitoring is possible, resulting in decreasing dismissals and enhancing patient care coordination. Advanced technologies are prompting automated healthcare systems. IoT devices are efficiently managing and tracking the resources for their better utilization. Using these techniques patients have the right to access their data remotely, and they can also set access permissions for the others [2].

DOI: 10.1201/9781003510932-1

The healthcare industry is experiencing a major change due to developments in technology. The traditional system of healthcare is transformed into smart healthcare utilizing IoT and blockchain. Smart healthcare improves patient monitoring, enhances working proficiency, and confirms the security of data [3].

1.1.1 Smart Healthcare

It includes online appointments, scheduling, billing, etc. Medical equipment occupancy can be checked through the use of IoT devices. Artificial intelligence (AI) can predict the behavior of diseases by utilizing the records of patients collected in the form of a dataset by the hospital. Through the use of mobile applications, medication reminders can be set to take medicine on time. Virtual reality is also helpful in maintaining smart healthcare, such as it can be used to provide professional training and can also be used in surgical simulation. Smart healthcare allows the patient to access their record sitting at home. Smart healthcare aims to influence technology and generate a more consistent, effective, and patient-centric healthcare ecology. By assimilating these technologies, healthcare professionals can progress diagnosis and management, improve patient involvement, and enhance resource division for better overall healthcare consequences, as shown in Figure 1.1.

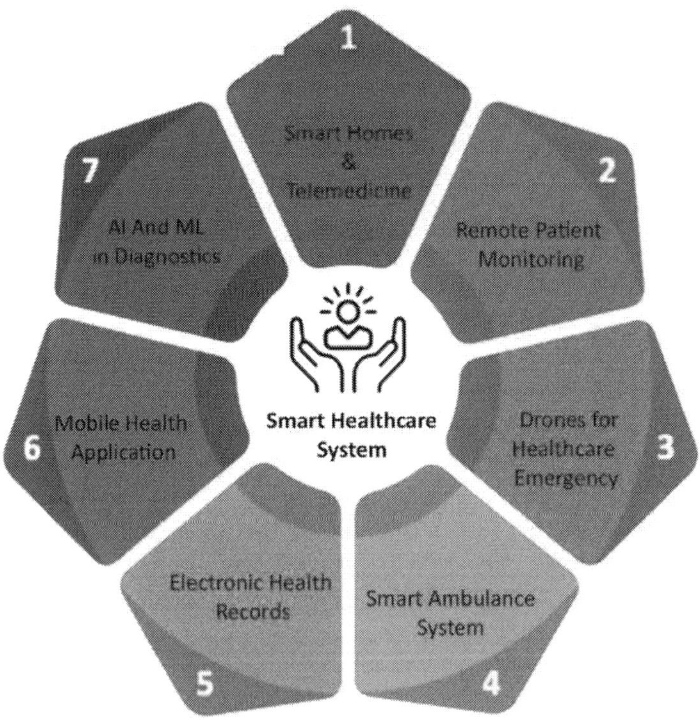

FIGURE 1.1 Smart healthcare system.

1.1.2 IoT

It refers to the interconnection of different types of devices to share information on the web. These devices contain sensors, actuators, and communication modules. These devices collect information and then share it with others on the web. For the working of IoT devices, an internet connection is required. The sensor collects the data and the actuator helps in decision-making. IoT devices process the data locally on the device itself and then transmit it to the server. This helps in reducing the latency and improves response time. To provide scalability data collected by the IoT devices can be transferred to clouds for further processing. The IoT devices are interoperable due to the support of various protocols [4]. These devices consume very less energy while working in integration.

Figure 1.2 represents the growth of wearable and portable IoT devices worldwide. The number of IoT devices is in the millions. The growth rate is very high as represented by the graph in the figure. The growth of these personalized IoT devices proved how remote monitoring could be used for smart healthcare management. Among the IoT devices used in Figure 1.2, the most widely used device is the insulin pump and the personal ECG is the least used IoT device.

1.1.3 Blockchain

Initially blockchain was developed for cryptocurrencies but these days it acts as a useful technique having significant applications in many fields like

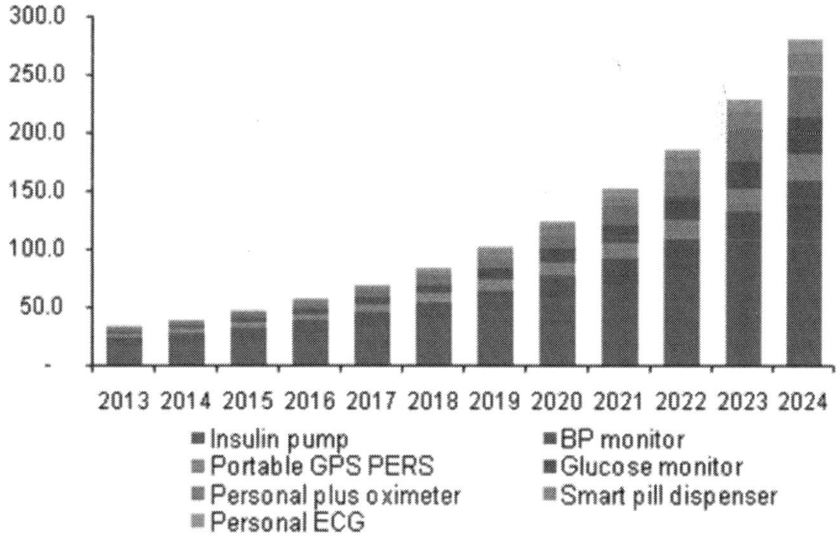

FIGURE 1.2 IoT healthcare devices growth (market growth of wearable IoT devices related to health). (Search images (bing.com).)

industries, medicine, education, banking, and many more. In healthcare, it plays an important role in handling the issues of data security and transparency [5]. The decentralized and non-changeable nature of blockchain guarantees that stored information is not modifiable and removable. Patients can access their records and can also set permissions for the others. The data stored on blockchain related to health is encrypted, which adds more security to the system. Only the authorized person can decrypt the data using the private key. It can be used to share health information among hospitals, doctors, labs, and insurance companies [6]. Figure 1.3 represents the basic structure of blockchain with its various features.

It can track the lifecycle of pharmaceuticals and medical materials, from manufacturing to delivery. This guarantees the authenticity of medicines and also decreases the risk of fake products, resulting in improved transparency in the supply chain. Blockchain can also be used for transparent insurance claims because of its immutable nature. It can be used to automate administrative processes by creating smart contracts; these contracts are self-executing with the terms of the agreement written into code. It could decrease the administrative load on healthcare workers and enhance efficiency.

Initially, blockchain implementation may demand high costs for establishment, but with its utilization in healthcare, costs get compromised due to its long-term services. Some of the features of blockchain are listed as follows:

- In blockchain, there is no central authority. It works on peer-to-peer networks.
- Everyone present in the network has access to all records, which results in high transparency.
- Blockchain has a public ledger that is accessible to all in the network.
- Once any transaction takes place, it cannot be modified later on.

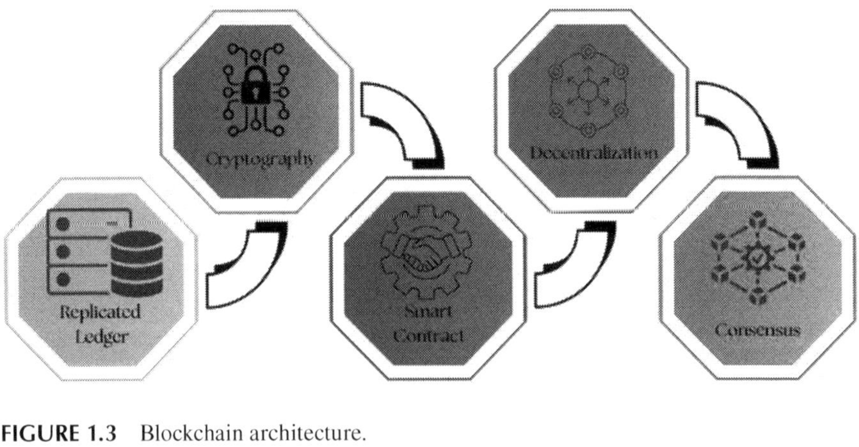

FIGURE 1.3 Blockchain architecture.

- All the transactions are secured using cryptography algorithms.
- It works on smart contracts and smart contracts are self-executing with the terms directly written on smart contracts code.
- No middleman is required for the execution of smart contracts.
- Transactions are very fast in blockchain. It works 24×7 without any disturbance.
- Every transaction is traceable in the blockchain.

1.2 LITERATURE REVIEW

Due to the advancement in technology, the healthcare industry is growing day by day. Healthcare daily activities use these techniques to fulfill the requirements of the patients. Onik et al. [7] reviewed papers related to the integration of IoT and blockchain for use in various healthcare applications. Papers from different datasets were collected for review. The papers were categorized based on their applications in the healthcare field. In the work the author mainly created six different types of applications. These six categories are remote patient monitoring, services related to medical, medical record maintenance electronically, detection of different types of disease, tracking of patients, tracking of medicine, and struggling with infectious diseases particularly COVID-19. The authors also listed the various issues that are associated with the integration of blockchain and IoT in healthcare technology. The authors also outlined some of the possible solutions for the integration of the same along with future scope.

IoT devices are highly utilized by healthcare professionals for collection of patient data. Then this collected data is processed and analyzed to identify the disease. The data may be misused by hackers so for the safety of data blockchain was applied by the authors. The decentralized and immutable nature of blockchain provides safety to the patient data. Ray et al. [8] integrated IoT and blockchain to make the healthcare system robust. These agreements are deliberated to support electronic healthcare record management. The data-flow design showed the integration of IoT and blockchain, named IoBHealth. The model was utilized for storing, processing, managing, and accessing healthcare data.

Dwivedi et al. [9] tried to resolve the issue of bandwidth and cost. They proposed a blockchain framework that was well-fitted for IoT devices. The proposed model has a distributed nature with the security of healthcare data. For security purposes, authors used cryptography algorithms during the transmission of data from one network to another network. IoT and blockchain-based remote health monitoring were proposed by Vahdati et al. [10]. In the proposed work, the authors reviewed various applications of healthcare based on the integration of IoT and blockchain systems. The remote monitoring health data was processed and analyzed by the authors. They proposed an IoT-blockchain-based model for finding solutions to the existing problems in the field like computational cost and security. Authors have done three case studies on the COVID-19 data for its storage and processing using some artificial techniques.

Blockchain in integration with IoT is used in many domains for electronic data management. IoT wearable devices efficiently collect real-time data from patients. The collected data is processed and analyzed to find any type of disease present. The early detection of disease means timely treatment of the disease. The problem of data security is resolved by blockchain technology. The maintenance of data is provided by blockchain technology along with the transmission of data from one network to another. Hemalatha [11] reviewed many papers based on the integration of these technologies. They tried to resolve the issue of data security on personal computers as well as on central servers. Srivastava et al. [12] provided a comprehensive literature review on blockchain technology for healthcare applications. The authors also listed the application of blockchain in healthcare. The authors also focused on COVID-19 data for its analysis. As the number of IoT devices is increasing day by day data collected is required to arrange and maintain along with security. The authors proposed applying AI and machine learning to collected data. Yogeshwar and Kamalakkannan [13] presented the issues related to the security of data. They also pointed out how security issues could be resolved using blockchain technology. Papers also provided analysis of blockchain-based security applications. IoT devices helped in collecting patient data and that data was used for remote health monitoring of patients.

At the time of COVID-19, tele-healthcare services played an important role in the life of the public. Tele-healthcare services help at the last moment for the people. The last moment of the patient resulted in a low risk of infection. The research work [14] proposed tele-healthcare laboratories where IoT devices were used to collect data on patients without any physical contact. The professionals like doctors, nurses, and staff helped each other through cloud services. Rathee et al. [15] generated the blockchain framework for the security of the health data of patients. Any change in data could be reflected by the blockchain model. Experimental results were compared with traditional approaches and it has been calculated that the proposed work achieved 86% high security of data against different types of attacks. Zaabar et al. [16] used blockchain technology for the security of healthcare data. They used the OrbitDB database with an Interplanetary File System (IPFS) and records were stored in a decentralized manner. The blockchain network was designed on Hyperledger fabric by using Hyperledger composer for storing hashes and data. The results were performed on Hyperledger Caliper. The comparison of the work proved robustness against attacks.

1.3 ROLE OF IOT DEVICES IN HEALTHCARE

Table 1.1 represents the role of wearable and portable IoT devices in smart healthcare. IoT devices play an important role in monitoring the health of patients remotely. With the help of IoT devices, we can measure the blood pressure, oxygen level, body temperature, and heart rate of the patient. These devices avoid the frequent general checkup of the patient.

TABLE 1.1
Role of IoT Devices in Smart Healthcare

Application	Sensor Used	IoT Role
Remote surgery	Surgical remote sensors	Data collection, management, and information passing using IoT devices.
Diabetes	IR sensors, CGM sensor	Low latency and high speed of advanced technologies allow for communication between patients and medical professionals.
Blood pressure	Raspberry Pi blood sensors, smartwatches, smart bands	IoT sensors collect the data and then high-speed communication technologies allow for data transmission without any delay to the concerned person.
Heartbeats	ECG sensors	High-speed Wi-Fi is required to transmit the data collected through IoT ECG sensors.
Remote rehabilitation	Wearable IoT sensors	Tracking of the patient and then reporting to the medical professional followed by feedback from a doctor is exchanged on time and securely due to high-speed technology.
Telemedicine	Different IoT sensors for monitoring health	Different wearable IoT sensors collect data of patients and based on the analysis of collected data, doctors suggest medicine to the patient.
Oxygen level	Oximeter	The level of oxygen is measured from time to time by the wearable IoT sensor and then data is shared with the medical person and they suggest if consultancy or medicine is required or not.
Skin cancer detection	Camera	The images taken by the camera are compared with the standard cancerous image to detect skin cancer. High-speed technology is a must for the detection of the same due to high throughput.
Injury analysis	Sensors for taking images from time to time	IoT devices can be used to take images of the injury at a fixed interval. Then recovery of the injury is checked by medical professionals and accordingly, they suggest medicine for recovery.
Eyes disorder	Camera	The images taken are compared with the standard images with some disorders. For the complete process cloud computing and edge computing techniques are used. The eye disorder can also be checked in real-time by the doctors utilizing video calls due to the good response time of high-speed technology.
Body temperature	Wearable IoT sensors for blood pressure	Smart IoT devices connected through high-speed technologies are very responsive due to low latency and high throughput.

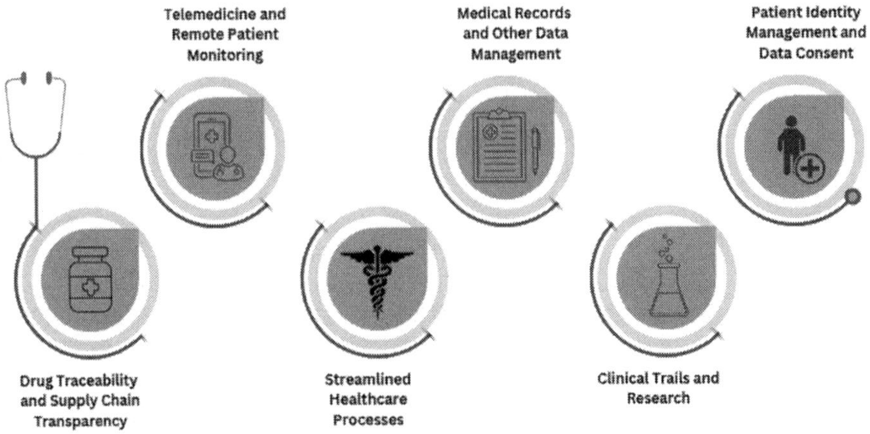

FIGURE 1.4 IoT-blockchain in smart healthcare.

1.4 INTEGRATION OF IOT-BLOCKCHAIN IN HEALTHCARE

Integration of IoT and blockchain with healthcare has the potential to transform the healthcare industry. The integration enhanced data security, patient care, resource utilization, easy operations, and many more. The immutable nature of blockchain ensures the integrity of healthcare data. As blockchain is decentralized it decreases the chance of data breaches. Blockchain works on smart contracts so the access rights are already automated resulting in authorized access to data. IoT devices can do continuous monitoring of the patient's health (glucose level, blood pressure, heart rate, and ECG) and this collected data can be used to do real-time analysis using blockchain. Figure 1.4 shows the integration of IoT and blockchain in smart healthcare.

Individual health patterns are identified using machine learning techniques on the collected data and then treatment can be planned [17]. The integration of these techniques improves interoperability as IoT devices collect from different sources and share this data using a blockchain protocol. IoT and blockchain can automate the task of billing, processing, and delivery by reducing manpower through smart contracts. Networks in blockchain can transfer large volumes of data with high speed.

1.5 ISSUES IN INTEGRATION OF IOT-BLOCKCHAIN IN HEALTHCARE

Some of the issues due to the integration of these techniques are listed as follows [18]:

- IoT devices are known for data collection. This collected data is processed through blockchain so transmission of data may be high because of the use of blockchain.
- Whether the data collected through IoT devices is accurate or not is very difficult.

- The data transfer in large amounts may result in network congestion.
- In blockchain, the memory required for data storage is high because each node contains information on all the transactions.
- There are no standards for the integration of IoT and blockchain with healthcare so transmission of information may cause issues.
- Strong technical expertise is required for the smooth synchronization of multiple devices.
- Smart contracts automate the process but it requires special knowledge in the field.
- Hardware and software demand increases as the overall cost of the system increases.
- Healthcare professionals are also required to train in the new technology. Blockchain records data immutability but it cannot ensure accuracy.

1.6 CONCLUSION

IoT and blockchain integration signify how healthcare data can be well managed and utilized. IoT helps in the collection of real-time data and blockchain provides security, transparency, and interoperability to the system. Blockchain works on smart contracts to automate the healthcare system. In this work, the author has provided basic details of the traditional healthcare system, and how the traditional healthcare system can be converted into a smart healthcare system by utilizing IoT and blockchain technology. Various applications of IoT devices and blockchain are discussed in the proposed work. Along with the merits of integration of these techniques, the demerits are also listed.

REFERENCES

1. Khan, A. A., Bourouis, S., Kamruzzaman, M. M., Hadjouni, M., Shaikh, Z. A., Laghari, A. A., … & Dhahbi, S (2023). Data security in healthcare industrial internet of things with blockchain. *IEEE Sensors Journal*, *23*(20), 25144–25151.
2. Sharma, A., Singh, M., Gupta, M., Sukhija, N., & Aggarwal, P. K. (2022). IoT and blockchain technology in 5G smart healthcare. In *Blockchain Applications for Healthcare Informatics* (pp. 137–161). Academic Press.
3. Chauhan, N., & Dwivedi, R. K. (2022, March). A secure design of the healthcare IoT system using blockchain technology. In *2022 9th International Conference on Computing for Sustainable Global Development (INDIACom)* (pp. 704–709). IEEE.
4. Pilania, U., Kumar, M., Singh, S., Adhalkha, P., & Satija, T. (2023, December). Securing confidential information on WhatsApp with blockchain technology. In *International Conference on Advancements in Smart Computing and Information Security* (pp. 53–61). Springer Nature Switzerland.
5. Pilania, U., Upadhyay, P., Tanwar, R., & Kumar, M. (2023). A creative domain of blockchain application: NFTs. In *Mobile Radio Communications and 5G Networks: Proceedings of Third MRCN 2022* (pp. 397–406). Springer Nature Singapore.
6. Azbeg, K., Ouchetto, O., Andaloussi, S. J., & Fetjah, L. (2022). A taxonomic review of the use of IoT and blockchain in healthcare applications. *Irbm*, *43*(5), 511–519.

7. Onik, M. M. H., Aich, S., Yang, J., Kim, C. S., & Kim, H. C. (2019). Blockchain in healthcare: Challenges and solutions. In *Big Data Analytics for Intelligent Healthcare Management* (pp. 197–226). Academic Press.
8. Ray, P. P., Dash, D., Salah, K., & Kumar, N. (2020). Blockchain for IoT-based healthcare: Background, consensus, platforms, and use cases. *IEEE Systems Journal, 15*(1), 85–94.
9. Dwivedi, A. D., Srivastava, G., Dhar, S., & Singh, R. (2019). A decentralized privacy-preserving healthcare blockchain for IoT. *Sensors, 19*(2), 326.
10. Vahdati, M., Gholizadeh HamlAbadi, K., & Saghiri, A. M. (2021). IoT-based healthcare monitoring using blockchain. In Applications of Blockchain in Healthcare (pp. 141–170). Springer.
11. Hemalatha, P. (2021). Monitoring and securing the healthcare data harnessing IOT and blockchain technology. *Turkish Journal of Computer and Mathematics Education (TURCOMAT), 12*(2), 2554–2561.
12. Srivastava, S., Pant, M., Jauhar, S. K., & Nagar, A. K. (2022). Analyzing the prospects of blockchain in the healthcare industry. *Computational and Mathematical Methods in Medicine, 2022*(1), 3727389.
13. Yogeshwar, A., & Kamalakkannan, S. (2021, May). Healthcare domain in IoT with blockchain-based security researcher's perspectives. In *2021 5th International Conference on Intelligent Computing and Control Systems (ICICCS)* (pp. 1–9). IEEE.
14. Celesti, A., Ruggeri, A., Fazio, M., Galletta, A., Villari, M., & Romano, A. (2020). Blockchain-based healthcare workflow for tele-medical laboratory in federated hospital IoT clouds. *Sensors, 20*(9), 2590.
15. Rathee, G., Sharma, A., Saini, H., Kumar, R., & Iqbal, R. (2020). A hybrid framework for multimedia data processing in IoT healthcare using blockchain technology. *Multimedia Tools and Applications, 79*(15), 9711–9733.
16. Zaabar, B., Cheikhrouhou, O., Jamil, F., Ammi, M., & Abid, M. (2021). HealthBlock: A secure blockchain-based healthcare data management system. *Computer Networks, 200*, 108500.
17. McGhin, T., Choo, K. K. R., Liu, C. Z., & He, D. (2019). Blockchain in healthcare applications: Research challenges and opportunities. *Journal of Network and Computer Applications, 135*, 62–75.
18. Yaqoob, I., Salah, K., Jayaraman, R., & Al-Hammadi, Y.(2022). Blockchain for healthcare data management: Opportunities, challenges, and future recommendations. *Neural Computing and Applications, 34*, 11475–11490.

2 Implementing Blockchain for Secure Medical Insurance Claim Settlement Process

Mrinal Pandey, Mamta Arora, and Prerna Kandpal

2.1 INTRODUCTION

Integrating blockchain technology into medical insurance claim settlements is a significant improvement for securely storing and sharing patient data. This change not only increases transparency but also builds trust among third-party administrators (TPAs), insurance companies, and patients. By tackling issues of data security and confidentiality, blockchain technology makes the claim settlement process more efficient and dependable.

Blockchain technology is essentially a decentralized system that records transactions on many computers, making it very difficult to change the records later without changing all the following records and getting agreement from the network. This makes blockchain very reliable and transparent, which is perfect for uses that need high trust and data accuracy. In medical insurance, blockchain ensures that information from documents like loan cards and Aadhaar cards is stored and sent securely. This is important because patient information is very sensitive and needs strong protection to prevent unauthorized access and breaches.

The literature underscores the significant potential of blockchain in revolutionizing the insurance industry. Blockchain enhances security and efficiency in insurance claim processing through smart contracts, ensuring transparent and immutable transaction records between patients and hospitals [1]. Also, blockchain enhances application security and transparency in the insurance claim process by using smart contracts for verification and consensus, thereby ensuring transaction integrity [2]. Previous studies highlight that blockchain helps manage data securely and in a decentralized manner, which also boosts system performance.

Using blockchain for settling insurance claims involves storing important information like Aadhaar numbers, PAN numbers, and invoices in smart contracts. This method keeps the data secure and makes it easy to access and manage. Smart contracts can handle many documents and patients, allowing the system to efficiently manage data for various patients overseen by different TPAs. Key functions in the smart contracts verify the existence of patients and TPAs, ensuring smooth interactions and data validation within the blockchain system.

DOI: 10.1201/9781003510932-2

Blockchain technology plays a crucial role in setting up access control rules that manage who can see and change data, ensuring that the information stays secure and reliable. This builds trust among all the users in the network because they know only authorized individuals can access certain data. Features like progress bars within the blockchain system let stakeholders see how far along document transfers are, improving transparency and accountability.

Patients also gain from using the blockchain system as it lets them track their documents within the network. By allowing patients to see the current status and location of their documents, the system not only makes things more transparent but also empowers patients to take an active role in managing their healthcare information.

Blockchain technology has the potential to transform the insurance industry [3]. It can be used to create a traceable online system for insurance claims, using blockchain and smart contracts. This system aims to automate claims settlement, securely verify customer identities, and reduce false claims through transparent information sharing. By integrating blockchain with electronic medical records (EMR), it ensures trust, reduces fraud, and improves customer service across various insurance sectors.

In conclusion, using blockchain in medical insurance claim settlement could revolutionize the industry by improving data security, transparency, and efficiency. The unchangeable and transparent nature of blockchain makes the insurance process more reliable and streamlined, benefiting everyone involved. Many studies support the use of blockchain in insurance, highlighting its potential to solve current problems and create a more secure and efficient future for medical insurance claims.

2.2 RELATED WORKS

The literature review by M. Thenmozhi et al. in [1] shows that blockchain technology has the potential to greatly improve how insurance claims are processed, making them more secure and efficient with the help of smart contracts. This idea uses blockchain to make health insurance claims more secure and streamlined, creating clear and unchangeable transaction records between patients and hospitals. Smart contracts automate the calculation of payments and verification, reducing mistakes and building trust. This method showcases how blockchain can provide secure and decentralized data management, enhance system performance, and address challenges like encryption and scalability in the insurance industry.

There exists a considerable body of literature by Dr. Jaideep Gera et al. in [2] on using blockchain technology to prevent fraud in insurance claims. This study suggests using IBM's blockchain platform to improve security and transparency in insurance applications. It describes how to implement this with involvement from the police, insurance companies, and agents, using smart contracts for verification. The study highlights blockchain's ability to ensure transaction integrity and prevent tampering with cryptographic signatures and unchangeable records. However, it mainly focuses on claim processing, and future research should explore scalability, security challenges, and integration with technologies like 5G. This could further improve the efficiency and fraud prevention capabilities of blockchain in the insurance industry.

It was reported in literature by Chin-Ling Chen et al. in [3] that blockchain and smart contracts could significantly change the insurance industry by improving efficiency, transparency, and security. This survey proposes an online system for insurance claims that uses these technologies to automate claim processing, securely verify customer identities, create industry blacklists, enhance mutual insurance, and combat fraud by sharing information openly. By combining blockchain with EMR and a strong Public Key Infrastructure (PKI), the system aims to transform insurance operations, ensuring trust, reducing fraud, and improving customer service across different types of insurance. Future developments are expected to expand blockchain's use in other areas of insurance.

This paper by Shraddha Arora et al. in [4] begins with a short review of the literature regarding the digitization of health insurance documents for cashless claim settlement using an intelligent document management system. The study looks at how natural language processing (NLP) and computer vision are used to extract information from various documents like hospital invoices, PAN cards, and Aadhaar cards. They highlight issues such as poor image quality and multilingual content, which require specific strategies to improve accuracy. The paper discusses the use of AI technologies like NLP and optical character recognition (OCR), which have shown high accuracy in document processing. However, it also mentions limitations, such as the lack of diverse datasets and ethical concerns with healthcare data, suggesting that future research should focus on including a wider range of documents and improving AI methods in medical claims processing.

A recent study by Nukala Poorna et al. in [5] concluded that blockchain technology offers promising solutions for connecting health insurance companies and hospitals. They pointed out current problems in the industry and suggested that blockchain could improve transparency, protect data better, and make processing insurance claims more efficient. They used Ethereum as the main platform and proposed a system using smart contracts to automate transactions and verify claims. Experiments with a prototype showed that this approach is feasible, which could lead to better cooperation and more efficient systems in the health insurance sector.

Jaya Kuckreja et al. in [6] used a practical approach, suggesting blockchain technology and InterPlanetary File System (IPFS) for a health insurance claim system. Their paper addressed issues of healthcare data security and fraud by proposing a model that increases transparency among insurers, hospitals, and insurance companies. They highlighted benefits like reducing fraud, speeding up claims processing, and enhancing transparency using smart contracts and secure data storage on IPFS. The study reviewed other blockchain applications in healthcare and emphasized system design, implementation steps, and testing methods, including smart contract integration and performance evaluation. Future research could focus on making the framework more scalable and integrating it with existing healthcare systems for further improvements.

Several studies, such as one conducted by Mohd. Nadeem and Shah [7], suggest that blockchain technology has the potential to significantly change the healthcare industry. Blockchain can be used to securely manage medical records, improve drug discovery and research, streamline clinical trials, detect medical fraud, and handle billing claims more efficiently. This technology offers strong security and transparency, with the help of smart contracts that automate processes and ensure accountability.

Research highlights blockchain's ability to enhance patient care and improve the management of healthcare data. Moreover, studies also explore how blockchain can secure patient data, improve communication between healthcare providers, and optimize medical workflows to increase efficiency and compliance. However, there are challenges to overcome, such as integrating blockchain with existing systems and achieving widespread adoption in the healthcare sector.

There exists a considerable body of literature by Leemore S. Dafny in [8] that discusses how combining companies in the private health insurance industry affects consumers. The study examines changes in premiums and other consumer outcomes due to consolidation. It also suggests ways to analyze potential impacts of future mergers. The research highlights the need for more data to understand whether consolidation benefits or harms consumers. By focusing on the health insurance sector, the study reviews existing literature and data on market structure and spending. It finds that consolidation generally leads to higher premiums and less competition. However, the study acknowledges limitations such as data biases and evolving healthcare policies. It recommends further research on the long-term effects of mergers and the policy implications, particularly under the Affordable Care Act.

Guy Zyskind et al. in [9] discuss the urgent issue of protecting user privacy when organizations collect centralized data. They explore both legal and technological approaches to safeguard personal information. Their study introduces concepts like openPDS frameworks and blockchain technology as potential solutions for secure and independent data management. They emphasize techniques such as data anonymization (for example, k-anonymity) and secure computation via openPDS. Future efforts are aimed at improving blockchain platforms to handle data more efficiently while ensuring confidentiality. However, challenges remain, including the inefficiency of current processing methods and concerns about how service providers retain data for future analysis.

It was reported in literature by Shuchih Ernest Chang et al. in [10] that adding blockchain technology to business process reengineering (BPR) can significantly change current centralized systems. Instead of completely redoing everything, this method focuses on improving efficiency and transparency by redesigning specific business processes. The research shows how blockchain can help move from centralized to distributed peer-to-peer systems, contributing new ideas to academic studies. Future research could explore blockchain's uses in fields like healthcare and supply chain logistics to create better overall systems. However, challenges such as scalability, compatibility between systems, and meeting regulations need addressing. Despite these challenges, integrating blockchain into BPR shows promise for improving how organizations innovate and operate.

Rutwik Senta et al. in [11] explored how blockchain technology can be applied in supply chain management (SCM) and logistics. They focused on improving visibility, tracking, and operational efficiency. The study suggested using the Polygon network blockchain to enhance traceability in the food supply chain. They proposed using smart contracts for governance and secure data storage to prevent tampering. To address cost issues and improve user experience, the research recommended integrating cloud services and account abstraction. This architectural approach aims to seamlessly connect Web2 and Web3 interfaces. Polygon's scalability was highlighted as beneficial for flexibility and interoperability with other blockchain systems. Overall, the research anticipates that these advancements could significantly enhance supply chain transparency, accountability, and public health.

2.3 BLOCKCHAIN

Blockchain technology is growing rapidly due to its decentralized nature, transparency, and immutable ledger system, as illustrated in Figure 2.1. Each transaction adds a new block to the blockchain network, forming a continuous chain linked through cryptographic hashes. This distributed ledger expands across a network of nodes, ensuring redundancy and resilience against data loss or manipulation. The decentralized architecture mitigates single points of failure, enhancing scalability and robustness as more participants join the network.

Blockchain ensures secure data storage through strong encryption and consensus mechanisms, as discussed in Section 2.3. Once stored, blockchain's immutability

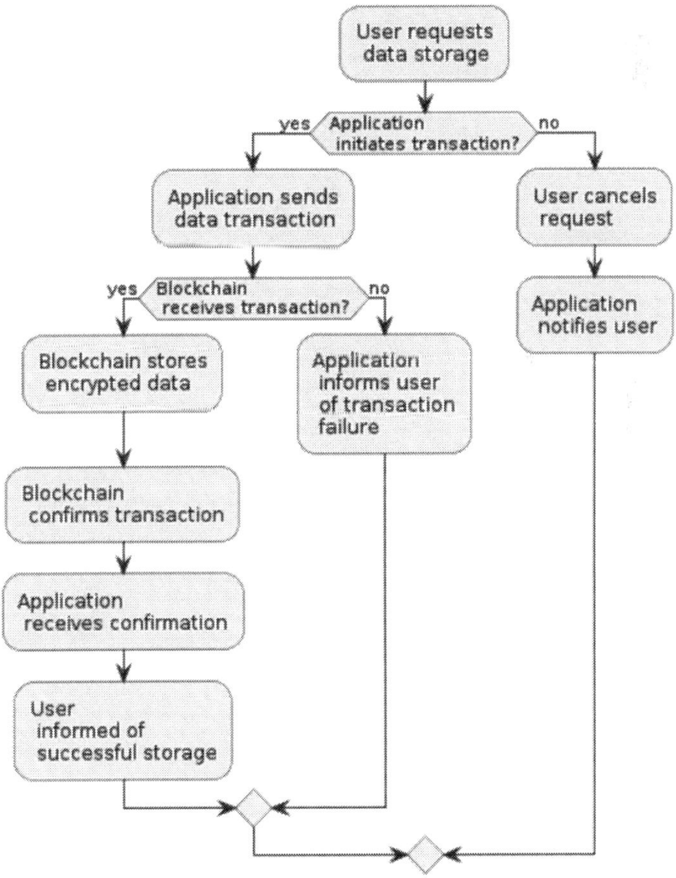

FIGURE 2.1 Blockchain data security flow.

prevents retroactive alterations, addressing concerns about tampering and fraud. Each block in the chain is linked by cryptographic hashes, ensuring data integrity and transparency across the network. This transparency is maintained through the decentralized nature of blockchain, where all transactions are recorded on a public ledger accessible to all participants. These features not only strengthen data security but also build trust among stakeholders by maintaining a dependable and verifiable record of transactions.

To implement best practices in secure data storage using blockchain, organizations should emphasize the encryption of sensitive data, utilize decentralized networks for data distribution across multiple nodes, and deploy robust consensus mechanisms such as proof of work or proof of stake. Regular audits and continuous monitoring of blockchain transactions are crucial for promptly detecting and responding to potential security threats. By adhering to these principles, blockchain technology enhances data security while fostering trust, transparency, and efficiency across various sectors, including finance and SCM.

2.4 PROPOSED METHODOLOGY

The proposed method involves using a strong blockchain system to securely store data. This system will be integrated with web applications to track medical insurance claims. It ensures that data remains reliable, transparent, and can grow as needed.

Figure 2.2 outlines a well-defined process designed for patients seeking medical insurance claims. Initially, users submit crucial documents, like PAN and Aadhaar, securely stored on the Polygon framework, renowned for its robust security measures within the Ethereum ecosystem. The subsequent stage involves sharing this data with TPAs,

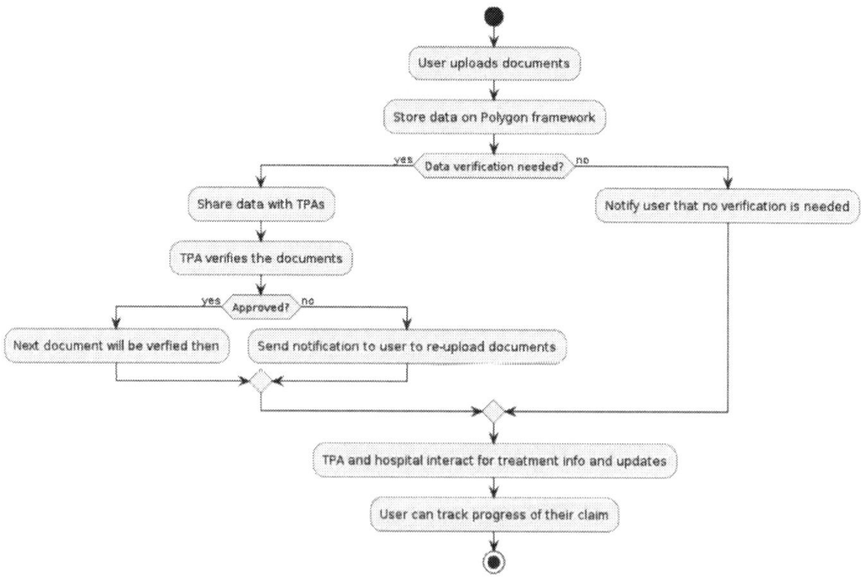

FIGURE 2.2 Working of model.

who possess restricted access for document verification. Upon approval of the documents, the process proceeds to the subsequent phase, enabling patients to track their claim progress in real time. Conversely, if the documents are not approved, patients promptly receive notifications prompting them to re-upload the necessary documentation.

Through this streamlined process, continuous interaction between TPAs and hospitals facilitates seamless exchange of precise treatment information and updates, ensuring a comprehensive approach to efficiently managing medical insurance claims.

2.4.1 Technologies Used

2.4.1.1 Web3

Web3 is the next evolution of the Internet, emphasizing decentralization and user control using blockchain technology. It allows for secure, transparent transactions without intermediaries, enhancing both security and transparency. In the model, Web3 technologies ensure secure, transparent transactions and interactions, allowing users to manage their data and transactions directly without intermediaries. This decentralization enhances the security and transparency of the medical insurance claim tracking system.

2.4.1.2 Polygon

Polygon is a Layer 2 solution for Ethereum that boosts transaction speeds and reduces costs. It makes blockchain applications more efficient and scalable, allowing more transactions at lower costs. By migrating the smart contracts to the Polygon network, the process benefits from increased efficiency and scalability. This allows the system to handle a higher volume of transactions at lower costs, making real-time tracking of medical insurance claims more feasible and cost-effective.

2.4.1.3 Smart Contracts and Ethereum

Smart contracts on Ethereum form the backbone of the data management system described. They enable automated execution of predefined terms and conditions, ensuring the secure storage and management of sensitive documents such as PAN and Aadhaar cards. Through smart contracts, data integrity is maintained, and processes like claim tracking can be automated, providing real-time updates to patients.

These technologies—Web3 for interface and interaction, Polygon for scalability, and Ethereum smart contracts for secure automation—combine to create a robust framework for implementing and overseeing blockchain-based solutions in healthcare and insurance sectors. This framework ensures improved efficiency, transparency, and greater user control over data and transactions.

2.4.2 Architecture of the Model

The model utilizes the technologies described in Section 2.4.2 to establish a well-structured architecture focused on secure data management and automated transactions.

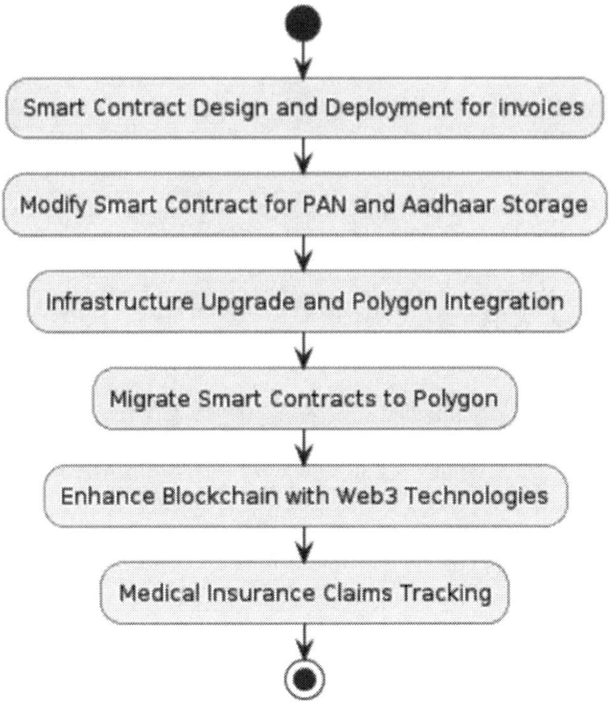

FIGURE 2.3 Architecture of framework.

The architecture described in Figure 2.3 outlines a systematic deployment of blockchain technologies, including Ethereum, Polygon, and Web3, specifically made for managing medical insurance claims. Initially, it focuses on developing and deploying initial smart contracts designed to securely store invoice data on the Ethereum blockchain, establishing a secure foundation for data management. Subsequent efforts enhance these contracts to include the secure storage of sensitive information like PAN and Aadhaar card details, ensuring their immutability through rigorous testing and validation processes.

Following this foundational phase, an infrastructure upgrade integrates Polygon as a scaling solution for Ethereum, aiming to improve transaction efficiency and reduce costs associated with the anticipated increase in transaction volumes from medical insurance claims. The migration of smart contracts to Polygon capitalizes on its scalability advantages, facilitating faster transaction processing. Concurrently, the architecture incorporates Web3 technologies to bolster blockchain functionalities, enhancing transaction security, transparency, and user control. These improvements play a critical role in enabling real-time tracking and monitoring of medical insurance claims, providing patients with timely updates on claim statuses.

In summary, this architectural approach establishes a robust framework for automating secure data management and transactions in the healthcare insurance sector. By strategically utilizing Ethereum, Polygon, and Web3 technologies, the architecture ensures operational efficiency, transparency, and an enhanced user experience throughout the management and tracking of medical insurance claims.

2.5 CONCLUSION

Blockchain technology in medical insurance claim settlements provides a strong solution for safekeeping and transferring data securely. With smart contracts, sensitive patient information like Aadhaar numbers, PAN numbers, and invoice data can be securely stored and accessed within the blockchain network. These smart contracts manage multiple documents and patients efficiently, ensuring smooth interactions and data validation among involved parties such as TPAs and insurance companies. Access control mechanisms bolster data security, while progress tracking features offer transparency and accountability during the claim settlement process. Ultimately, blockchain builds trust among stakeholders by enabling real-time data verification and enhancing transparency in insurance claims.

2.6 FUTURE WORK

Future research will aim to make the blockchain system better at handling more data and transactions in medical insurance. The integration with other systems and adding new technologies like Internet of Things devices for real-time data tracking could be addressed. The access to data can be improved and be more controlled to make it more secure and create easier ways for everyone involved to use the system.

ACKNOWLEDGMENTS

This research is part of a funded project titled "Medical Claim Settlement using BlockChain Technology". We acknowledge our sincere gratitude to IBITF for providing funds and support for this project development.

REFERENCES

1. M. Thenmozhi, R. Dhanalakshmi, S. Geetha, and R. Valli, "Withdrawn: Implementing Blockchain Technologies for Health Insurance Claim Processing in Hospitals," *Mater. Today Proc.*, Mar. 2021, doi: 10.1016/j.matpr.2021.02.776.
2. J. Gera, A. R. Palakayala, V. K. K. Rejeti, and T. Anusha, "Blockchain Technology for Fraudulent Practices in Insurance Claim Process," in *2020 5th International Conference on Communication and Electronics Systems (ICCES)*, Coimbatore, India: IEEE, Jun. 2020, pp. 1068–1075. doi: 10.1109/ICCES48766.2020.9138012.
3. C.-L. Chen, Y.-Y. Deng, W.-J. Tsaur, C.-T. Li, C.-C. Lee, and C.-M. Wu, "A Traceable Online Insurance Claims System Based on Blockchain and Smart Contract Technology," *Sustainability*, vol. 13, no. 16, Art. no. 16, Jan. 2021, doi: 10.3390/su13169386.
4. S. Arora, M. Pandey, M. Arora, K. Gupta, V. Sharma, and L. Nagpal, "Digitization of Health Insurance Documents for The Cashless Claim Settlement Using Intelligent Document Management System," *Procedia Comput. Sci.*, vol. 235, pp. 1319–1331, Jan. 2024, doi: 10.1016/j.procs.2024.04.125.

5. N. Poorna, P. V. Sravan, K. Baruah, S. S. Mudigonda, and P. Krihsna, "Use of Blockchain Technology in integrating Heath Insurance Company and Hospital," 2018. Accessed: Jun. 22, 2024. [Online]. Available: https://www.semanticscholar.org/paper/Use-of-Blockchain-Technology-in-integrating-Heath-Poorna-Sravan/b4f8c01c4f3d43780a0cfde502e5b2b6a9082553
6. J. Kuckreja, P. Nigde, and P. Patil, "Health Insurance Claim Using Blockchain," *Int. Res. J. Eng. Technol.*, vol. 08, no. 05, pp. 2406–2409, 2021.
7. M. Nadeem and D. Shah, "Pre Settlement in Insurance for Hospital Treatment Using Cryptocurrency and Blockchain Technology," *Int. J. Res. Eng. Sci. Manage.*, Oct. 2021, Accessed: Jun. 22, 2024. [Online]. Available: https://journal.ijresm.com/index.php/ijresm/article/view/1460
8. L. S. D. Dafny, "Evaluating the Impact of Health Insurance Industry Consolidation: Learning from Experience," Commonwealth Fund, New York, NY United States, Nov. 2015. doi: 10.15868/socialsector.25054.
9. G. Zyskind, O. Nathan, and A. Pentland, "Decentralizing Privacy: Using Blockchain to Protect Personal Data," IEEE Conference Publication, IEEE Xplore, Accessed: Jun. 22, 2024. [Online]. Available: https://ieeexplore.ieee.org/abstract/document/7163223
10. S. E. Chang, Y.-C. Chen, and M.-F. Lu, "Supply Chain Re-Engineering Using Blockchain Technology: A Case of Smart Contract Based Tracking Process," *Technol. Forecast. Soc. Change*, vol. 144, pp. 1–11, 2019, doi: 10.1016/j.techfore.2019.03.015.
11. R. Senta, A. Sawant, and S. Jain, "Enhancing Food Safety and Transparency in the Supply Chain Through Polygon Blockchain and Cloud Integration," *Int. J. Comput. Digit. Syst.*, vol. 16, no. 1, pp. 189–202, May 2024, https://journal.uob.edu.bh/handle/123456789/5673

3 Challenges of IoT-Based Healthcare Ecosystem and Possible Remedies

Shakeel Ahamad, Ratneshwer Gupta, Garima Jain, Deepak Uprety, and Sovers Singh Bhist

3.1 INTRODUCTION

The Internet of Things (IoT) is a renowned instance of the new era of possibilities brought about by the convergence of healthcare and technology. The IoT-based healthcare ecosystem is promising to revolutionize patient care, clinical operations, and medical research; however, amid the transformative potential lie myriad challenges that impede its seamless integration and realization of its full benefits.[1] This chapter delves into the multifaceted challenges encountered within the IoT-based healthcare landscape. It proposes actionable remedies to address these hurdles, fostering a more robust and resilient future for healthcare delivery.

In recent years, the proliferation of connected devices and advancements in data analytics and Artificial Intelligence (AI) have propelled the healthcare industry toward a paradigm shift.[2] The IoT, a network of linked devices that gather, share, and analyze data, is the leader of this revolution and has the potential to completely redefine the way healthcare is delivered. By seamlessly integrating devices, sensors, and systems, IoT enables real-time monitoring, remote patient management, personalized treatment plans, and predictive analytics, enhancing patient outcomes, optimizing resource utilization, and driving efficiencies across the care continuum.[3]

Nevertheless, there are many obstacles to fully utilizing IoT in healthcare, necessitating cautious navigation and creative solutions. These challenges span technological, regulatory, ethical, and operational realms, each presenting unique complexities and barriers to adoption. In this chapter, we elucidate the key challenges confronting the IoT-based healthcare ecosystem and explore possible remedies to overcome these impediments, paving the way for a more resilient and transformative healthcare landscape.[4]

The diverse array of connected devices and sensors in IoT-enabled healthcare engenders interoperability issues, data silos, security vulnerabilities, and scalability concerns.[5] Fragmented systems and incompatible protocols hinder seamless data exchange and integration, impeding the development of cohesive healthcare solutions. Moreover, the sheer volume and velocity of healthcare data generated exacerbate data management, storage, privacy, and cybersecurity

DOI: 10.1201/9781003510932-3

challenges. To mitigate these technological challenges, concerted efforts are needed to standardize protocols, promote interoperability, enhance data security measures, and invest in robust infrastructure capable of accommodating exponential data growth.

The highly regulated nature of the healthcare industry, coupled with stringent data privacy and security standards, poses significant compliance challenges for IoT deployments. Adherence to HIPAA (Health Insurance Portability and Accountability Act) regulations and GDPR (General Data Protection Regulation) necessitates meticulous attention to data governance, consent management, encryption, and audit trails. Additionally, navigating the complex landscape of regulatory approvals and certifications for medical devices and software further complicates the deployment and adoption of IoT solutions.[6] Addressing these regulatory hurdles requires collaboration between stakeholders, regulatory bodies, and policymakers to establish clear guidelines, streamline compliance processes, and foster a conducive regulatory environment for innovation in healthcare.

The rest of the chapter is organized as follows. Section 3.2 discusses the future technological challenges of IoT devices in healthcare. Finally, the conclusion is given in Section 3.3.

3.2 CHALLENGES IN IoT-BASED HEALTHCARE

The integration of IoT in healthcare raises profound ethical and societal considerations about patient privacy, consent, autonomy, and equitable access to care. Concerns regarding data ownership, consent management, algorithmic bias, and the commodification of health data underscore the need for ethical frameworks and governance mechanisms to safeguard patient rights and mitigate potential harm. Furthermore, discrepancies in digital literacy and access to technology deepen the already-existing healthcare disparities by increasing the digital divide and aggravating differences in health outcomes. Addressing these ethical and societal implications requires a holistic approach prioritizing transparency, inclusivity, and patient-centered care in designing, deploying, and evaluating IoT-based healthcare solutions.[7]

The convergence of healthcare and technology has ushered in a new era of possibilities, transforming the landscape of patient care and clinical operations. The IoT, a network of linked devices that gather, share, and analyze data, is at the pioneering of this revolution and has the potential to completely redefine the way healthcare is delivered.[8] While IoT holds immense potential for enhancing patient outcomes, optimizing resource utilization, and driving efficiencies across the care continuum, its widespread adoption is accompanied by technological challenges. In this section, we delve into the future technological challenges anticipated in the IoT-based healthcare ecosystem and explore potential remedies to address these hurdles, ensuring a resilient and transformative future for healthcare delivery.[9] Figure 3.1 represents major components of the smart healthcare system.

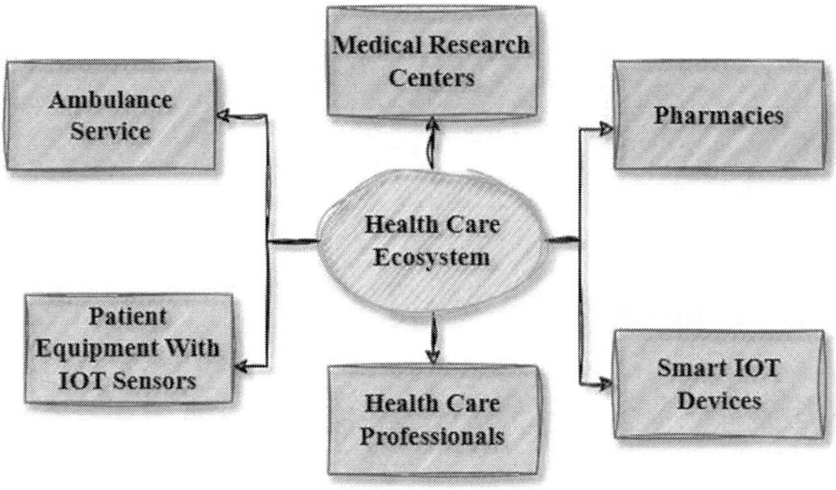

FIGURE 3.1 Healthcare ecosystem components.

3.2.1 Interoperability and Data Integration

One of the fundamental technological challenges facing IoT-based healthcare ecosystems is interoperability and data integration. As the number of connected devices and sensors proliferates, healthcare organizations face a heterogeneous landscape of devices operating on disparate protocols and standards. This fragmentation impedes seamless data exchange and integration, resulting in data silos and inhibiting the development of comprehensive healthcare solutions.[10] Figure 3.2 represents the interoperability of smart healthcare systems with the use of IoT devices.

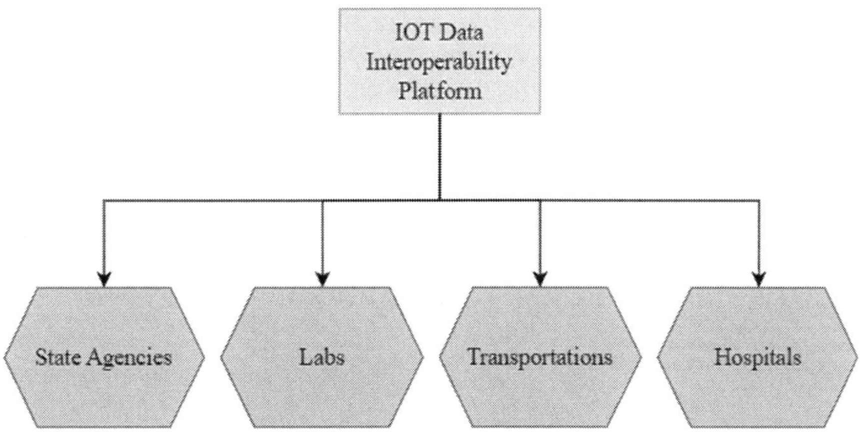

FIGURE 3.2 Interoperability platform for IoT-based smart healthcare.

Healthcare has long struggled with fragmented patient information systems, hindering seamless data synchronization. While integration tools have improved data sharing, questions arise about their impact on patient care. Are healthcare providers adequately informed about patient treatment and outcomes? Challenges remain in aligning semantics across systems and integrating cloud-based electronic medical records (EMRs). Interoperability, crucial for effective data exchange, faces delays and interruptions.[11]

3.2.1.1 Remedies

3.2.1.1.1 Standardization Efforts

Collaborative initiatives to standardize communication protocols and data formats can facilitate interoperability among diverse IoT devices. Organizations such as the Institute of Electrical and Electronics Engineers (IEEE) and the International Organization for Standardization (ISO) have a major role in the creation and promotion of interoperability standards for the IoT in the healthcare industry.[12]

3.2.1.1.2 Middleware Solutions

Implementation of middleware platforms that serve as intermediaries between disparate devices and systems can facilitate data translation, protocol conversion, and seamless integration. Middleware solutions offer a layer of abstraction, enabling interoperability without requiring extensive modifications to existing infrastructure.[13]

3.2.1.1.3 API-Driven Integration

Adopting Application Programming Interfaces (APIs) allows healthcare organizations to create standardized data exchange and interoperability interfaces. Organizations can facilitate seamless integration with third-party applications and platforms by exposing APIs for accessing and manipulating data.[14]

3.2.1.1.4 Blockchain

Blockchain promises secure, real-time access to patient data. Deloitte Consulting suggests blockchain could revolutionize healthcare, enhancing security and interoperability. Industry observers see blockchain as a tool to address healthcare challenges, potentially fostering transparent, value-based care. As healthcare evolves, technology, including blockchain, plays a vital role in shaping a more efficient and interconnected healthcare ecosystem (Figure 3.3).[15]

3.2.2 Scalability and Resource Constraints

As IoT deployments in healthcare continue to scale, organizations face scalability and resource constraint challenges. The exponential growth in the volume and velocity of healthcare data generated by connected devices strains existing infrastructure, leading to performance bottlenecks, latency issues, and resource contention. Moreover, the proliferation of edge computing devices at the network periphery

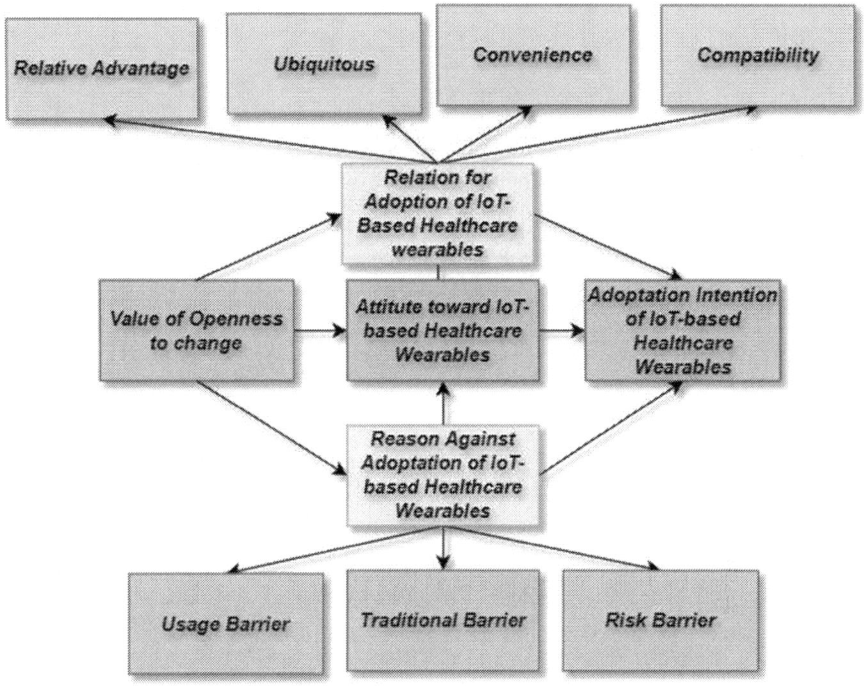

FIGURE 3.3 Conceptual framework for adoption of IoT-based healthcare wearables.

exacerbates resource constraints, necessitating efficient resource allocation and management strategies.[16]

3.2.2.1 Remedies

Edge Computing Paradigm: Embracing edge computing paradigms allows healthcare organizations to distribute computational tasks closer to the data source. Consequently, less bandwidth and delay are needed. To improve scalability and reduce the load on centralized infrastructure, edge computing allows real-time data processing at the network edge.[17]

Cloud-Based Solutions: Leveraging cloud-based platforms and services provides healthcare organizations with scalable infrastructure and on-demand resources to accommodate fluctuating workloads. Cloud computing offers elastic scaling capabilities, allowing organizations to dynamically provision and deprovision resources based on demand, optimizing resource utilization.[8] Figure 3.4 represents the use of IoT in healthcare from various perspectives.

Resource Optimization Algorithms: Developing resource optimization algorithms and intelligent workload management strategies can enhance resource utilization efficiency in IoT-based healthcare ecosystems. To anticipate resource demand, machine learning algorithms can evaluate past data trends. This allows for proactive resource allocation and mitigating performance bottlenecks.[18]

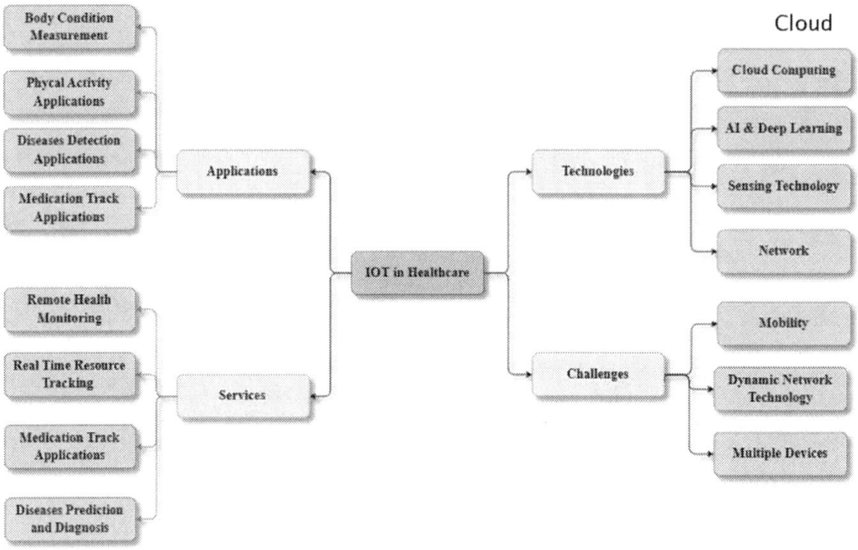

FIGURE 3.4 IoT in healthcare: Applications, services, technologies, and challenges.

3.2.3 Data Security and Privacy

In IoT-based healthcare ecosystems, where sensitive patient data availability, confidentiality, and integrity are critical, security and privacy issues pose serious hurdles. Because IoT devices are interconnected and healthcare data is ubiquitous, they are vulnerable to various security risks, such as ransomware events, malware assaults, and unauthorized access. Furthermore, due to legislative requirements, healthcare businesses are subject to strict obligations to protect patient information and maintain compliance with data protection standards.[19]

3.2.3.1 Remedies

End-to-End Encryption: Implementation of end-to-end encryption mechanisms ensures that data remains encrypted throughout its lifecycle, mitigating the risk of unauthorized access and interception. Healthcare organizations can safeguard patient confidentiality and protect sensitive information from unauthorized disclosure by encrypting data at rest, in transit, and in use.[20]

Identity and Access Management (IAM): Healthcare businesses may prevent illegal access to IoT devices and healthcare systems by enforcing granular access controls and authentication processes by deploying comprehensive identity and access management solutions. IAM solutions make it easier to manage user identities, rights, and permissions centrally, ensuring that only people with the proper authorization can access resources and sensitive data.[21]

Security-by-Design Principles: Adopting security-by-design principles entails integrating security considerations into designing, developing, and implementing IoT-based healthcare solutions. By prioritizing security from the outset and implementing security controls at every architecture layer, healthcare organizations can proactively mitigate security risks and vulnerabilities.[22]

3.2.4 Reliability and Resilience

The reliability and resilience of IoT-based healthcare systems are critical considerations, particularly in mission-critical applications where downtime or service interruptions can have severe consequences for patient safety and care delivery. Ensuring the continuous availability and uptime of IoT devices and systems requires robust infrastructure, fault-tolerant architectures, and proactive monitoring and management practices.[23]

3.2.4.1 Remedies

3.2.4.1.1 Redundancy and Failover Mechanisms

Implementing redundancy and failover mechanisms at both the hardware and software levels enhances system resilience and mitigates the impact of hardware failures, network outages, and service disruptions. In the case of a failure, minimal downtime is experienced because of automated failover techniques, replicated databases, and redundant components that guarantee system continuation.[24]

Healthcare businesses can proactively detect and resolve possible problems before they become severe breakdowns by implementing continuous monitoring and predictive maintenance procedures. Combining predictive analytics and machine learning algorithms with real-time device performance metrics monitoring makes identifying abnormalities and system health degradation easier early on, enabling prompt intervention and preventive maintenance.[25]

Creating thorough planning for disaster recovery and business continuity is crucial to minimizing the effects of significant occurrences like cyberattacks, natural disasters, and infrastructure breakdowns. To guarantee that patient care and service delivery continue in an emergency, healthcare companies must set up comprehensive backup and recovery protocols, alternative communication routes, and contingency plans.[26]

3.2.5 Challenges and Issues in IoT Healthcare

The development of safe and effective data collection techniques for IoT healthcare monitoring systems remains a challenge despite the potential advantages of IoT for enhancing human health. This section examines several open research issues: functionality, performance, data privacy, dependability, security, and stability.

3.2.5.1 Security and Privacy

Security and privacy raise several ethical issues. Hackers can easily access electronic health records that are kept on cloud servers and have been digitally converted. Hackers may get access to patient medical data due to a security breach on the cloud server. The misuse of health information, data protection regulations, data ownership, and user authentication are all impacted by this. Enhancing trust in IoT use in healthcare requires addressing security and privacy issues in IoT system design and development. To lower security risks and safeguard privacy, security protocols must be implemented at every IoT layer and component.

For users to rely on sensors, devices, gateways, and IoT services while protecting their identity, privacy, and safety, developers must make sure that IoT "things" and the systems they connect to are secure. These security and privacy concerns are often overlooked when developing personal and commercial technologies. Integrated security techniques, including wireless transceivers and hardware and software components for sensors, impact several health-related IoT remote monitoring applications. To protect user privacy during data storage and transfer, applications that gather data from several sensors and devices employ robust authentication, encryption, and other security mechanisms.

These apps frequently have privacy restrictions and link with already-existing healthcare data. They might still require the most recent data security protocols to be included. To protect their privacy, people should be able to determine who is legally permitted to see and alter their data. Users of the IoT need to have faith that their data will be handled safely and responsibly. Remote monitoring is essential given the possible secondary uses for the data collected by house IoT. Remote health monitoring is one way that users of these systems can get their data. Figure 3.5 represents key challenges in the IoT healthcare system.

Protecting privacy and data security continues to be a significant obstacle to the health of IoT. Spied or modified data delivered to the data-processing unit may lead to an imprecise big data analysis. Securing the data transfer from the nodes to the processing unit is essential. Throughout processing, the confidentiality of the data supplier must also be maintained.

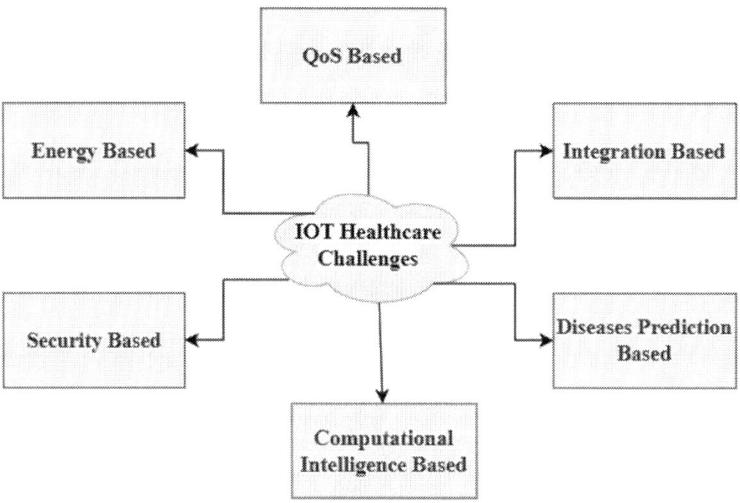

FIGURE 3.5 Key challenges in IoT healthcare.

3.2.5.2 Quality of Service

Quality of service (QoS) is the protection of a certain level of data transmission performance with a changeable priority that varies according to requirements. The primary challenge in data transmission from the end node to the server node is maintaining the confidentiality of critical patient information. The time it takes for a data packet to be delivered between node devices is known as IoT latency. QoS indicators apply to every sub-component of the IoT architecture, ranging from the cloud services used for healthcare to an individual's home. To make sure there are no memory leaks or improperly cached data, memory consumption needs to be monitored.[27]

The results are poor signal, sluggish network speeds, abrupt disconnection or inconsistent connectivity, and delays and interruptions to data transfer caused by wireless disruption. Another performance parameter is energy consumption management, which can reduce functionality, stability, performance, and dependability. The constant gathering of data from devices uses a lot of energy. After a depletion period, the battery requires time to recharge; however, the gadget cannot monitor constantly during this time. A low battery on the smartphone may cause a symptom like wireless interference.[28]

When the wireless sensor nodes do not receive enough power to function, a severe problem arises. More must be done to enable the nodes to run on the least amount of electricity to produce green energy, renewable technology, and energy-efficient solutions. Patients who need round-the-clock medical monitoring can now live at home instead of in a hospital thanks to the IoT. Wearable technology, however, may make some individuals uncomfortable. Noise may be produced during data transfer from the sensor to the monitoring center and control unit. When the design is better, data can be transported with the least amount of integrity loss. Using noise removal techniques can help improve data streams.[29]

Most techniques now in use for ECG monitoring call for guided signal analysis, which adds costs and raises the possibility of detection errors. Signal analysis with machine learning can save expenses and increase productivity. The price of medical services is another factor; therapeutic equipment is now more crucial than ever. Researchers must engage in more excellent discourse and work to reduce the expenses linked to IoT healthcare systems. The high cost of monitoring equipment is one major issue facing the IoT healthcare system. IoT still needs to make affordable treatment services available to the public.[30]

Medical equipment is becoming more and more expensive. Device designers, manufacturers, evaluators, and testers must solve these problems without compromising cost or quality to improve consumers' impressions and experiences with such expensive goods. If the problems can be resolved, IoT in the healthcare sector will improve.[31]

3.2.5.3 Computational Intelligence

It is still in the early days of computational intelligence technology. To improve consumers' impressions and experiences of such expensive products, device developers, producers, assessors, and testers must solve these problems without compromising quality or price. If the problems are resolved, the prospects for IoT in the healthcare sector are bright. To optimize data, networks, and traffic appropriately, computation on the IoT-based healthcare monitoring systems is done on edge devices. These services are connected to data collection, calculation, and evaluation related to the Internet. On the other hand, we must recognize edge devices' restricted processing power and resource capabilities.[32]

3.2.5.4 Integration

Integrating current instruments or devices with external technologies ensures data accuracy and consistency throughout their existence and prepares them for future expansion. Unresolved issues still plague the integrity of the data. When expanded upon and combined with other external devices that provide many advantages, IoT-based monitoring systems will improve quality of life. Integration tool development will significantly impact communications, processing, and integration-related services. Expanding the IoT healthcare monitoring systems would require adopting new or related technologies like the cloud and software-defined network (SDN).[33]

3.2.5.5 Energy

The battery life of IoT devices used in the healthcare industry that depend on monitoring is limited. These devices use energy even when not explicitly needed to read sensors and operate in energy-saving mode. The device must do some tasks even in energy-saving mode, but its power supply is constrained.[34] Many medical devices, particularly wearables and devices for patients who require continuous health monitoring, are perpetually dependent on batteries. Long-term monitoring requires an ideal system that combines power-efficient hardware architecture with low-power communications. Reduced power consumption is a fascinating new field of application made possible by activity-aware energy models. Context-aware episodic sampling can improve performance from poor to excellent.[35]

3.2.5.6 Disease-Prediction

The IoT facilitates early disease detection in fitness programs, aids in diagnosing and treating ailments, especially chronic diseases, and supports elder care. The advancement of healthcare that can detect a patient's disease early will be advanced by expanding the planned system. This disease-prediction technology can help doctors treat patients as soon as possible by reducing the time it might take to identify an ailment. This will all come from better medical services, improved results for the healthcare sector, and decreased medical costs (such as needless lab and X-ray exams). As a result, developing a low-cost, standalone system that monitors crucial metrics, transmits information to the cloud or NLP, and swiftly notifies patients for their benefit is also required.[36]

3.2.6 Suggestions and Recommendations

To solve the communication challenges and weaknesses of previous studies, wearable healthcare devices must be enhanced and combined with other developing technology developments, considering the limitations of current research. Researchers must ensure that any suggested technologies are safe, adaptable, and simple to maintain a satisfied clientele. Integrating wearable sensors into healthcare systems presents new disease management and healthcare prospects. By linking sensors and health-tracking devices to the cloud for round-the-clock monitoring, the IoT can offer a solution.[37]

Instant access to and security for health records are provided via the server. Future development of a system to diagnose COVID-19 and chronic illness in patients could aid medical professionals in making the best decisions and improving patient outcomes.[38] This could enhance the functionality of IoT-based healthcare systems by combining several technological advancements. AI, fog computing, SDNs, big data, the Internet of Nano-Things (IoNT), and the Tactile Internet (TI) are some examples of these integration strategies. Sensor data can yield valuable and reliable discoveries when AI is integrated with IoT-based healthcare monitoring systems. Processing power could be moved closer to the point of need with the help of the fog/edge idea.[39]

Big data computing can be applied to the IoT healthcare monitoring systems because it can efficiently manage massive amounts of data. Future technology developments like SDNs, the Internet of Next Things (IoT), and the TI may further enhance IoT-based healthcare systems by increasing their capabilities and usefulness.[40]

3.3 CONCLUSION

In conclusion, while the IoT-based healthcare ecosystem holds immense promise for transforming care delivery, addressing the inherent challenges is imperative to realize its full potential. By proactively addressing technological, regulatory, ethical, and societal hurdles, stakeholders can collaboratively pave the way for a resilient and patient-centric healthcare future. IoT serves as an enabler of innovation, efficiency, and improved health outcomes.

IoT-based healthcare has enormous potential to transform clinical operations, patient care, and medical research in the future. However, to fully realize this promise, several technological obstacles must be overcome, ranging from interoperability to scalability to security and dependability. Healthcare businesses may overcome these obstacles and clear the path for a resilient and transformational future by taking a proactive stance and putting corrective measures like standardization initiatives, edge computing paradigms, encryption techniques, and resilience plans into place. Stakeholders may leverage the IoT to improve patient outcomes, optimize resource usage, and drive efficiency across the healthcare continuum, eventually advancing care delivery in the digital age by working together and embracing innovation.

The IoT can enhance healthcare in a plethora of ways. These consist of lower costs and higher performance, accuracy, and efficiency. Optimizing healthcare systems through automation is now feasible because of the advantages of the IoT. Future workers in the sector will find this work introductory as it provides a thorough reference guide on IoT and healthcare monitoring systems. This work reviews and thoroughly examines the current literature on IoT-based health monitoring systems. Besides doing a literature analysis, the study provides comprehensive information regarding their significance and benefits. Along with a taxonomy of health monitoring sensors and a discussion of wearables in healthcare systems, we also address the difficulties and unresolved problems with security, privacy, and QoS. Future research directions have also been suggested.

REFERENCES

1. Elhoseny M, Ramírez-González G, Abu-Elnasr OM, Shawkat SA, Arunkumar N, Farouk A. Secure Medical Data Transmission Model for IoT-Based Healthcare Systems. *IEEE Access*. 2018;6:20596–20608. doi:10.1109/ACCESS.2018.2817615
2. Al-Atawi AA, Khan F, Kim CG. Application and Challenges of IoT Healthcare System in COVID-19. *Sensors*. 2022;22(19):1–21. doi:10.3390/s22197304
3. Selvaraj S, Sundaravaradhan S. Challenges and Opportunities in IoT Healthcare Systems: A Systematic Review. *SN Applied Sciences*. 2020;2(1):1–8. doi:10.1007/s42452-019-1925-y
4. Jaime FJ, Muñoz A, Rodríguez-Gómez F, Jerez-Calero A. Strengthening Privacy and Data Security in Biomedical Microelectromechanical Systems by IoT Communication Security and Protection in Smart Healthcare. *Sensors (Basel)*. 2023;23(21). doi:10.3390/s23218944
5. Ahmed S, Khan M. Securing the Internet of Things (IoT): A Comprehensive Study on the Intersection of Cybersecurity, Privacy, and Connectivity in the IoT Ecosystem. *AI, IoT and the Fourth Industrial Revolution Review*. 2023;13(9):1–17. https://scicadence.com/index.php/AI-IoT-REVIEW/article/view/13
6. Allioui H, Mourdi Y. Exploring the Full Potentials of IoT for Better Financial Growth and Stability: A Comprehensive Survey. *Sensors*. 2023;23(19). doi:10.3390/s23198015
7. Giannaros A, Karras A, Theodorakopoulos L, Karras C, Kranias P, Schizas N, et al. Autonomous Vehicles: Sophisticated Attacks, Safety Issues, Challenges, Open Topics, Blockchain, and Future Directions. *Journal of Cybersecurity and Privacy*. 2023;3(3):493–543. doi:10.3390/jcp3030025
8. Kim S, Kim S. User Preference for an IoT Healthcare Application for Lifestyle Disease Management. *Telecomm Policy*. 2018;42(4):304–314. doi:10.1016/j.telpol.2017.03.006
9. Wang X, Wu Y. *Fog-Assisted Internet of Medical Things for Smart Healthcare*. Vol 69; 2023. doi:10.1109/TCE.2023.3253896
10. Mohammed BG, Hasan DS. Smart Healthcare Monitoring System Using IoT. *International Journal of Interactive Mobile Technologies*. 2023;17(1):141–152. doi:10.3991/ijim.v17i01.34675
11. Suryanarayana G, Prakash K LNC, Ansari MD, Gunjan VK. IOT for Healthcare. *Internet of Things*. 2024; Part F1851(2):201–218. doi:10.1007/978-3-031-09955-7_12
12. Rao AS, Sreeja Mole SS, Jagan D, Ramesh R. Navigating the Internet of Things (IoT): Towards a Smart and Sustainable Future – Opportunities, Issues and Challenges. *International Journal of Early Childhood Special Education*. 2023;15(4):20–31. doi:10.48047/intjecse/v15i4.4
13. Kodali RK, Swamy G, Lakshmi B. An Implementation of IoT for Healthcare. *2015 IEEE Recent Advances in Intelligent Computational Systems, RAICS 2015*. Published online 2016:411–416. doi:10.1109/RAICS.2015.7488451
14. Chibuike MC, Grobbelaar SS, Botha A. Overcoming Challenges for Improved Patient-Centric Care: A Scoping Review of Platform Ecosystems in Healthcare. *IEEE Access*. 2024;12(November 2023):14298–14313. doi:10.1109/ACCESS.2024.3356860
15. Marengo A. Future of AI-Driven IoT: Identifying Emerging Trends in Intelligent Data Analysis and Privacy Protection. *Preprints.org*. Published online 2024: 202312.2184.v3. doi:10.20944/preprints202312.2184.v3
16. Adel A. Future of Industry 5.0 in Society: Human-Centric Solutions, Challenges and Prospective Research Areas. *Journal of Cloud Computing*. 2022;11(1). doi:10.1186/s13677-022-00314-5

17. Imran M, Zaman U, Imran, Imtiaz J, Fayaz M, Gwak J. Comprehensive Survey of IoT, Machine Learning, and Blockchain for Health Care Applications: A Topical Assessment for Pandemic Preparedness, Challenges, and Solutions. *Electronics (Switzerland).* 2021;10(20):1–37. doi:10.3390/electronics10202501
18. Curado M, Madeira H, da Cunha PR, Cabral B, Abreu DP, Barata J, Roque L, Roger I. Internet of Things. *Cyber Resilience of Systems and Networks.* 2020; 8(July 2016):381–401. http://link.springer.com/10.1007/978-3-319-77492-3_16
19. Raskar C, Nema S. A Review on Internet of Things (IoT) in Healthcare. *International Journal of Applied Engineering Research.* 2016;11(20):479–484.
20. Abdulmalek S, Nasir A, Jabbar WA, Almuhaya MAM, Bairagi AK, Khan MAM, et al. IoT-Based Healthcare-Monitoring System towards Improving Quality of Life: A Review. *Healthcare (Switzerland).* 2022;10(10). doi:10.3390/healthcare10101993
21. Li C, Wang J, Wang S, Zhang Y. A Review of IoT Applications in Healthcare. *Neurocomputing.* 2024;565(October 2023):127017. doi:10.1016/j.neucom.2023.127017
22. Chander B, Gopalakrishnan K. *Security Vulnerabilities and Issues of Traditional Wireless Sensors Networks in IOT.* Vol 174; 2019. doi:10.1007/978-3-030-33596-0_21
23. Birje MN, Hanji SS. Internet of Things Based Distributed Healthcare Systems: A Review. *Journal of Data, Information and Management.* 2020;2(3):149–165. doi:10.1007/s42488-020-00027-x
24. Shaikh TA, Rasool T, Verma P. Machine Intelligence and Medical Cyber-Physical System Architectures for Smart Healthcare: Taxonomy, Challenges, Opportunities, and Possible Solutions. *Artificial Intelligence in Medicine.* 2023;146(October):102692. doi:10.1016/j.artmed.2023.102692
25. Skarmeta AF, Santa J, Martinez JA, Parreira JX, Barnaghi P, Enshaeifar S, et al. IoTCrawler: Browsing the Internet of Things. *2018 Global Internet of Things Summit, GIoTS 2018.* Published online 2018. doi:10.1109/GIOTS.2018.8534528
26. Suryandari Y. Survei IoT Healthcare Device. *Jurnal Sistem Cerdas.* 2020;3(2):153–164. doi:10.37396/jsc.v3i2.55
27. Khan MA. Challenges Facing the Application of IoT in Medicine and Healthcare. *International Journal of Computations, Information and Manufacturing (IJCIM).* 2021;1(1):39–55. doi:10.54489/ijcim.v1i1.32
28. Rohokale VM, Prasad NR, Prasad R. A cooperative Internet of Things (IoT) for rural healthcare monitoring and control. *2011 2nd International Conference on Wireless Communication, Vehicular Technology, Information Theory and Aerospace and Electronic Systems Technology, Wireless VITAE 2011.* Published online 2011. doi:10.1109/WIRELESSVITAE.2011.5940920
29. Alashlam L, Alzubi A. Taxonomic Exploration of Healthcare IoT: Challenges, Solutions, and Future Frontiers. *Applied Sciences.* 2023;13(22):12135. doi:10.3390/app132212135
30. Popoola O, Rodrigues M, Marchang J, Shenfield A, Ikpehia A, Popoola J. A Critical Literature Review of Security and Privacy in Smart Home Healthcare Schemes Adopting IoT & Blockchain: Problems, Challenges and Solutions. *Blockchain: Research and Applications.* Published online 2023:100178. doi:10.1016/j.bcra.2023.100178
31. Sarathkumar R, Tahsien A-Q. Navigating the Future of the Internet of Things: Emerging Trends and Transformative Applications. *Babylonian Journal of Internet of Things.* 2023;2023:8–12. doi:10.58496/bjiot/2023/002
32. Chaterji S, Naghizadeh P, Alam MA, Bagchi S, Chiang M, Corman D, et al. Resilient Cyberphysical Systems and their Application Drivers: A Technology Roadmap. Published online 2019:1–36. http://arxiv.org/abs/2001.00090
33. Bansal S, Kumar D. AI and IoT in Smart Healthcare. *AI for Big Data-Based Engineering Applications from Security Perspectives.* Published online 2023:21–43. doi:10.1201/9781003230113-2

34. Pradhan B, Bhattacharyya S, Pal K. IoT-Based Applications in Healthcare Devices. *Journal of Healthcare Engineering* 2021;2021. doi:10.1155/2021/6632599
35. Adam M, Hammoudeh M, Alrawashdeh R, Alsulaimy B. A Survey on Security, Privacy, Trust, and Architectural Challenges in IoT Systems. *IEEE Access.* 2024;12(April):57128–57149. doi:10.1109/ACCESS.2024.3382709
36. Alansari Z, Soomro S, Belgaum MR, Shamshirband S. The Rise of Internet of Things (IoT) in Big Healthcare Data: Review and Open Research Issues. *Advances in Intelligent Systems and Computing.* 2018;564:675–685. doi:10.1007/978-981-10-6875-1_66
37. Alabdulatif A, Thilakarathne NN. Bio-Inspired Internet of Things: Current Status, Benefits, Challenges, and Future Directions. *Biomimetics.* 2023;8(4):1–29. doi:10.3390/biomimetics8040373
38. Dhinakaran D, Sankar SMU, Selvaraj D, Raja SE. Privacy-Preserving Data in IoT-based Cloud Systems: A Comprehensive Survey with AI Integration. Published online 2024. http://arxiv.org/abs/2401.00794
39. Ishaq K, Shah Farooq S. Exploring IoT in Smart Cities: Practices, Challenges and Way Forward. arXiv preprint arXiv:2309.12344.
40. Alkurdi AAH, Zeebaree SRM. Navigating the Landscape of IoT, Distributed Cloud Computing: A Comprehensive Review. *Academic Journal of Nawroz University.* 2024;13(1):360–392. doi:10.25007/ajnu.v13n1a2011

4 Securing AI in Healthcare

Innovations, Architectures, and Privacy Solutions

Amanjot Kaur and Rohit Tanwar

4.1 INTRODUCTION

Artificial intelligence (AI) is a field of computer science that gives machines ability to perform various activities with intelligence comparable to humans [1]. AI applications can be found in many fields, including banking, healthcare, manufacturing, and construction [2]. It is rapidly being used in AI-based remote surgeries in healthcare sector. AI in healthcare involves the use of Machine Learning (ML) algorithms to analyse and collect complex data. ML techniques, such as deep learning, computer vision, robotics, and Natural Language Processing (NLP), are utilized in healthcare sector [3]. These algorithms identify behaviour patterns and create logic to provide well-defined output to end users. ML is a powerful tool for predicting and understanding huge amounts of healthcare data.

AI helps healthcare industry by identifying and preventing diseases. It is utilized in a wide range of healthcare applications, such as patient monitoring facilities, pharmaceutical research, diagnosis, and medication. In healthcare industry, electronic health record (EHR) helps to collect historical data for purpose of disease prevention and diagnosis. Several medical institutions have developed AI algorithms for their departments, including The Mayo Clinic and Memorial Sloan Kettering Cancer Centre [4]. IBM and Google have also developed AI algorithms to support operational initiatives at lower costs. It enhances patient care and staff needs in healthcare sector [5]. AI integration in healthcare enhances diagnosis, treatment plans, and patient care. But still, security and privacy challenges are considered a major issue in healthcare industry [6]. However, this book chapter explores AI in healthcare sector; it highlights advantages and privacy concerns. This work aims to explore how AI can improve predictive analytics and diagnostics. Additionally, it discusses necessity to address privacy and security standards in healthcare to mitigate current security problems. The chapter's organizational structure is shown in Figure 4.1.

DOI: 10.1201/9781003510932-4

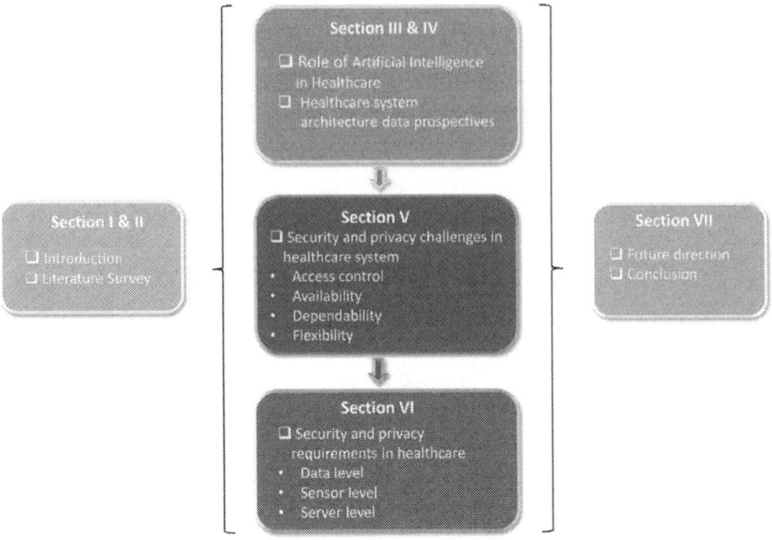

FIGURE 4.1 Structure of the paper.

4.2 RELATED WORK

Several approaches have been proposed using AI in healthcare sector. Most of researchers have explored AI in healthcare by combining various techniques, but there is a lack of significant efforts in analysing secured AI in healthcare. These issues include data privacy and protection, medical device security, incident prediction, data encryption, integrity and secure authentication. For instance, to assess performance metrics like scalability, accuracy, and malware attacks on wearable technology, Alabdulatif et al. [7] propose an AI-based secure architecture. However, further work needs to enhance security and privacy of AI and blockchain-based intelligent healthcare systems to completely address multiple security risks, such as buffer overflow, masquerade, clone phishing, and phone phishing. Adnan et al. [8] highlight issues with privacy and security that are related to various healthcare applications. Herein, authors cover many approaches to provide safe, privacy-protecting ML for medical applications. Alshehri et al. [9] evaluate edge-intelligent smart healthcare research on Internet of Things (IoT), whereas IoMT focuses on 2014–2020 journal publications, examining topics like edge computing, security, medical signal fusion and AI.

Ghazal et al. [10] present an IoT-AI system for healthcare security, which uses wireless sensor networks to monitor and secure patient information. For ensuring personalized access, it offers a single-user interface for record management. In comparison to alternative approaches, simulation research shows high rates of data delivery and transmission. Additionally, it also enhances throughput, efficient bandwidth monitoring, energy consumption, and performance rates. Zaman et al. [11] examine how IoT and AI technology can be used in healthcare to fulfil industry's expanding needs. Herein, authors examine developments regarding these novel paradigms. Additionally, authors also focus on security, functionality, and the development of enabling technology.

Albahri et al. [12] explore prior research based on explainable robots, digital health, blockchain, forecasting, decision support, and transparency. Additionally, it provides current key evaluations while demonstrating dependability. It looks at the feasibility of implementing reliable AI apps in healthcare industry. Moreover, in this study methodology for enhancing AI security is also emphasized by using random and unique secret keys. Almalawi et al. [13] improve medical professionals' access to patient-sensitive data stored on a cloud-based system. Herein, authors enhance privacy standards and reduce the amount of time needed to encrypt and decrypt data. Patil et al. [14] highlight advantages of AI, such as personalized medicine, clinical decision support systems, and workflow optimization. These AI-enabled applications are used to improve healthcare outcomes. It highlights the necessity of ethical issues, including patient privacy and data security.

Elnawawy et al. [15] provide a case study that illustrates how malicious data points introduced during inference compromise a diabetic monitoring system. More interestingly, authors demonstrate how an attacker can exploit vulnerability in Bluetooth communication pipeline linking ML-enabled app and glucose monitor. However, it demonstrates cutting-edge techniques for risk assessment to identify and evaluate these novel threats. This study emphasizes need to develop methods for assessing the security of AI-powered health devices. Stilinski et al. [16] explore challenges and opportunities in IoT networks for federated learning. The authors here provide important methodologies for ensuring data security and integrity. It designs algorithms for optimizing model training across heterogeneous devices. Table 4.1 shows various AI-enabled techniques that have been applied in healthcare sector.

TABLE 4.1
Summary AI Techniques in Healthcare

Sr. No.	Authors, Year of Publication	Technique Used	Findings	Limitations
1	Qayyum et al. (2020) [8]	Different deep learning as well as ML-methodologies.	Examine privacy and security issues in several healthcare application areas and provide possible solutions for safe and data-protecting AI and ML in the field of medicine.	While this study examines many techniques to improve security and privacy, there is a lack of sufficient attention to issues that arise when applying stated techniques to actual healthcare systems.
2	Alshehri et al. (2020) [9]	IoT and IoMT	Explores IoT- and IoMT-based edge-intelligent smart healthcare, focusing on journal publications on medical signal fusion, edge computing, AI, and security.	There is a lack of awareness of recent advancements and trends in smart healthcare and technology.

(Continued)

TABLE 4.1 *(Continued)*
Summary AI Techniques in Healthcare

Sr. No.	Authors, Year of Publication	Technique Used	Findings	Limitations
3	Ghazal et al. (2021) [10]	AI systems, Internet of Things, and IoT-AIS.	IoT-AIS uses wireless sensor networks to monitor and encrypt patient data, which improves performance, reduces delay estimates, allows bandwidth monitoring, and increases security for the healthcare industry.	Fails to address potential scalability issues and practical obstacles of integrating IoT-AIS systems in large hospitals.
4	Zaman et al. (2022) [11]	blockchain, Internet of Things, and AI	Investigate the application of IoT and AI in healthcare, focusing close attention on their progress, security, and performance to address growing concerns.	It does not concentrate on a thorough examination of the advantages and difficulties associated with combining blockchain, IoT, and AI in a healthcare setting.
5	Albahri et al. (2023) [12]	AI	Investigates the viability and possible methodological improvements of AI in healthcare, with a focus on blockchain, digital health, predictability, assistance with decisions, and explainable robotics.	Lack of attention on how AI is now affecting healthcare sector.
6	Almalawi et al. (2023) [13]	Serpent (LRO-S)-based healthcare system with Lionized Remora Optimization.	By employing random, unique secret keys, organizations can lower the time it takes to encrypt and decode data stored in cloud, strengthen privacy standards, and make it more affordable for healthcare providers to access patient-sensitive data.	It doesn't give a thorough analysis of how LRO-S encryption approach stacks up against other encryption strategies in medical contexts.
7	Patil et al. (2023) [14]	AI	Highlights ethical issues and explores advantages of AI, such as clinical decision support systems and personalized medicine, to investigate its potential to improve healthcare outcomes.	It doesn't include details about certain measurements or assessment techniques.
8	Elnawawy et al. (2024) [15]	AI	Highlights the need for enhanced risk analysis methods for AI-powered medical devices, citing a recent attack on an ML-enabled glucose monitoring system.	It doesn't apply its conclusions to other kinds of ML-enabled medical systems; instead, it concentrates on a particular case study.

4.3 ROLE OF AI IN HEALTHCARE

In healthcare sector, AI is widely applied for many different applications, such as disease treatment, medicine, patient monitoring, disease prediction, and disease prevention [17]. Figure 4.2 illustrates how AI is being used in healthcare sector. AI is a preventative strategy that aids in the identification and prediction of various types of disease. Its foundation lies in gathering previous data from EHRs to prevent and diagnose diseases. This data is then used for different types of disease prediction and treatment purposes. Moreover, AI obtains this data through the use of conventional medical procedures like X-rays [18]. More interestingly, robotics is used by AI in the development of medications and surgery. Currently, healthcare industry is experiencing exponential development in research due to possibilities of present AI research [19]. Over next five years, the US government is set to allocate over $2 billion towards AI-related healthcare sectors, such as radiology, psychiatry, dermatology, screening, and medication interactions [20].

4.3.1 Radiology

Application of AI in radiology departments has significantly increased during the last few years. AI is being utilized in radiology to diagnose and identify diseases through technologies like computerized tomography (CT) and Magnetic Resonance Imaging (MRI) [20]. However, AI algorithms in radiology can enhance accuracy and recall of identifying pneumonia in patients compared to non-participant radiologists [21]. AI is expected to lead to shorter consultation times and increased concurrent patient visits in radiography.

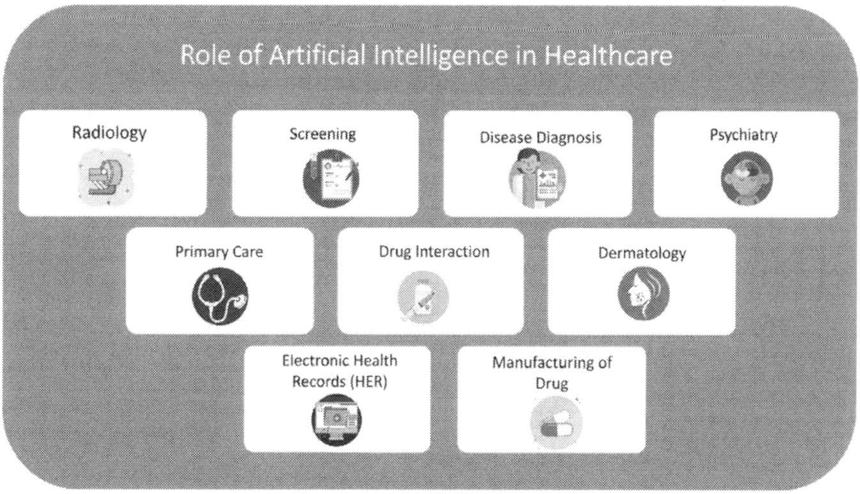

FIGURE 4.2 Role of Artificial Intelligence in healthcare.

4.3.2 Screening

Use of AI in radiology departments has significantly increased in the last several years. Radiology is utilizing AI to diagnose disorders through technologies like CT and MRI [22].

4.3.3 Psychiatry

AI applications are currently in proof-of-concept stage; they are being utilized to study depression and anxiety. However, Facebook implemented screening for suicidal thoughts. Healthcare professionals have several professional, ethical, and regulatory concerns about these kinds of applications [23].

4.3.4 Primary Care

AI technologies are increasingly utilized in primary care for predictive modelling, business analytics, and decision-making support [24].

4.3.5 Disease Diagnosis

AI technologies like support vector machines, decision trees, and neural networks are rapidly being utilized in healthcare sector to identify various diseases. AI is significantly enhancing diagnostic capabilities of doctors through the integration of Medical Learning Classifiers (MLCs) and EHRs [25].

4.3.6 Dermatology

Deep learning has significantly enhanced the effectiveness of dermatology as an imaging modality in image processing. Moreover, deep learning and dermatology are closely associated with healthcare industry [26]. On the other hand, deep learning and AI methodology have revolutionized dermatology in terms of image-processing strategy. Image-processing strategy makes it more efficient and basic than other outdated methods. Figure 4.3 illustrates three primary image processing methods in dermatology.

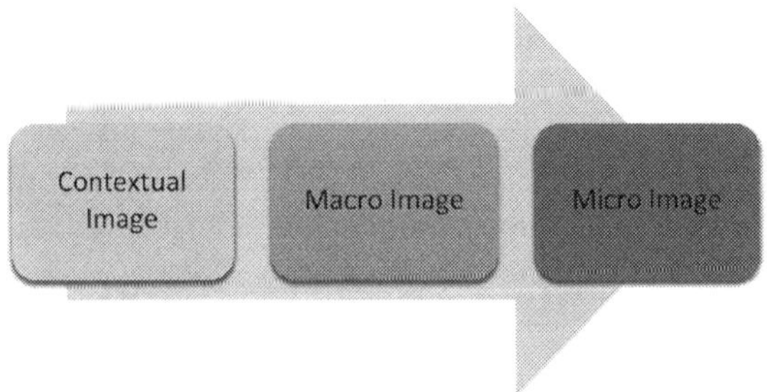

FIGURE 4.3 Distinct image processing.

Moreover, AI in image processing is being used in face photography to identify keratinocyte skin cancer. Additionally, dermatology-level classification of skin cancer can be established using decaying pictures. Similarly, skin cell recognition can be achieved with a microscope and a neural network [27].

4.3.7 Drug Interaction

NLP has the potential to enhance AI algorithms in healthcare by identifying drug interactions and reducing patient dosages. However, ML and deep learning techniques extract potential causes and consequences [28].

4.3.8 Manufacturing of Drugs

The process of creating new drugs has also become quicker and simpler because of AI. Moreover, AI is a medicine molecule that helps to treat Obsessive-Compulsive Disorder (OCD). It is a disorder that has not been effectively treated with traditional methods for around five years [29].

4.3.9 Electronic Health Records

Advancement of healthcare technology is largely driven by EHRs and AI. It improves disease information and record interpretation in healthcare sector. NLP aids in medication record preparation, clinician data analysis, and identifying common conditions like myocardial infarction and heart attack. However, AI algorithms estimate disease death probabilities based on patient and family data [30]. More interestingly, brain-computer interface is poised to revolutionize healthcare sector by providing significant benefits to disabled individuals and those with spinal cord injuries [31]. However, utilizing advanced AI-based technologies can effectively treat issues like cancer, chronic illnesses, and risk assessment [32, 33].

4.4 HEALTHCARE SYSTEM ARCHITECTURE DATA PERSPECTIVES

Healthcare data warehouse architecture is a complex framework that governs the design of data warehouses. Healthcare organizations consider factors, such as size, goals, and specialization area, before selecting a data warehouse design [34]. However, organizations should consult healthcare data warehouse suppliers before selecting an architectural model. The healthcare sector primarily utilizes individual and enterprise data warehousing architectural models. Figure 4.4 shows the structure of healthcare data warehouse.

4.4.1 Individual Data Warehousing

Individual data warehouses are also known as individual data marts. These are architectural models that integrate various subsets of data stored in data warehouses. This architecture focuses on a specific functional area within a healthcare organization [35]. However, a data mart can be seen as an isolated digital data repository.

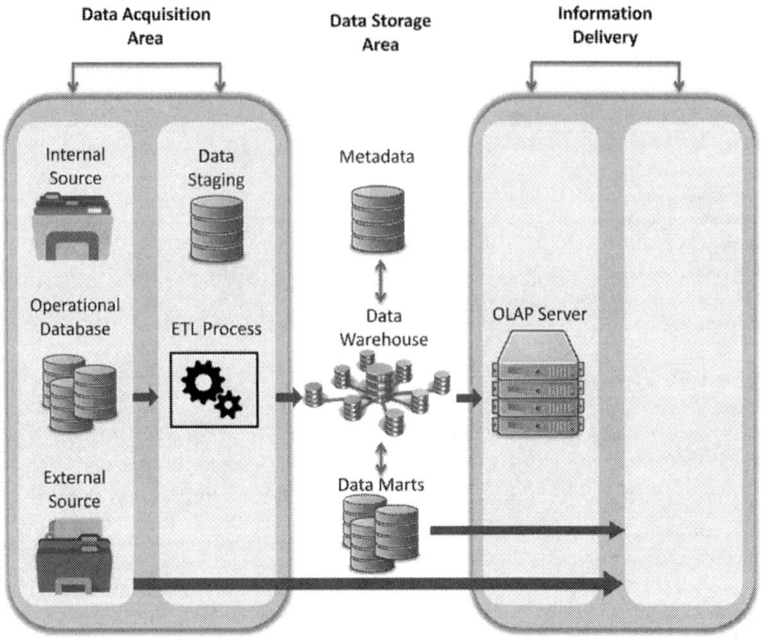

FIGURE 4.4 Healthcare data warehouse architecture.

Essentially, a data warehouse is a simplified version of a data warehouse designed for specific departments or divisions within an organization. Moreover, these disciplines include radiological technology, pharmacy, and outpatient care [36]. Healthcare organizations with a single data centre can analyse specific data, like rare diseases, and make necessary progress.

4.4.2 Data Warehousing

The healthcare data warehouse offers healthcare providers a comprehensive alternative for storing and analysing large volumes of data from several sources. The architectural model, as depicted in Figure 4.5, consists of four layers.

a. *Data Source Layer*: Data from various internal and external sources related to research activity are included in data source layer. However, hospital data can be gathered from various sources, including clinical sources, ERPs, EMRs/EMRs, pharmacy management platforms, lab websites, and insurance claim processing software, surveys, polls, and CRM systems [37].
b. *Staging Layer*: Staging layer is also known as staging zone. It temporarily manages a large overflow of erroneous data from the data source layer. Moreover, ETL method is utilized for data aggregation, anonymity, and normalization operations [38].
c. *Data Storage Layer*: In healthcare data warehousing architecture, this layer serves as the foundation. A cloud, SQL, or hybrid database is a

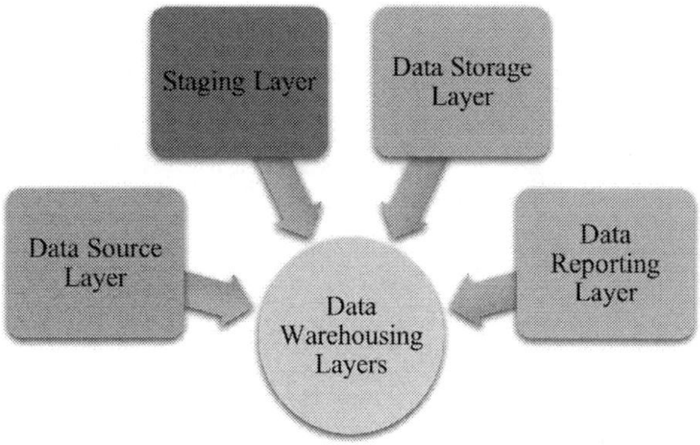

FIGURE 4.5 Data warehousing architecture.

storage system for terabytes of structured data, loaded via ETL/ELT procedures, and left for analysis. However, storage layers can support independent data marts. An enterprise data warehouse offers significant benefits for healthcare industry, including dependent and hybrid models. More interestingly, it is recommended to organize and store data at this layer into separate data warehouses, as long as it is accessible to other healthcare departments [39].

d. *Data Reporting Layer*: This layer is also referred to as a business intelligence layer. It enables integration of data lake technologies, ML, and analytical toolkits with external applications. Moreover, this final layer evaluates relevant data using statistical analysis, data mining, visualizations, graphs, charts, and report summaries [40].

4.5 SECURITY AND PRIVACY CHALLENGES IN HEALTHCARE SYSTEMS

The healthcare sector is undergoing significant transformation due to increasing use of AI in healthcare applications [41]. However, medical data is being used to train AI to find trends. It is utilized to understand the relationship between diagnosis and treatment. AI is transforming healthcare by enhancing patient experiences and medical care.

As healthcare AI advances, privacy concerns must be addressed. Moreover, data security safeguards need to be established and maintained. The development underscores the critical role of AI in healthcare for its reliability, safety, and effectiveness in delivering optimal patient care and outcomes [42]. The difficulties with privacy and security in healthcare are shown in Figure 4.6.

a. *Access Control*: Limiting and controlling authorized users' access to resources is known as access control. The system identity, authorization, and authentication are subject to three distinct security and privacy criteria. Identification is a crucial aspect of user authentication, but it is not necessarily a security concern. However, as a result, it is employed to modify the user

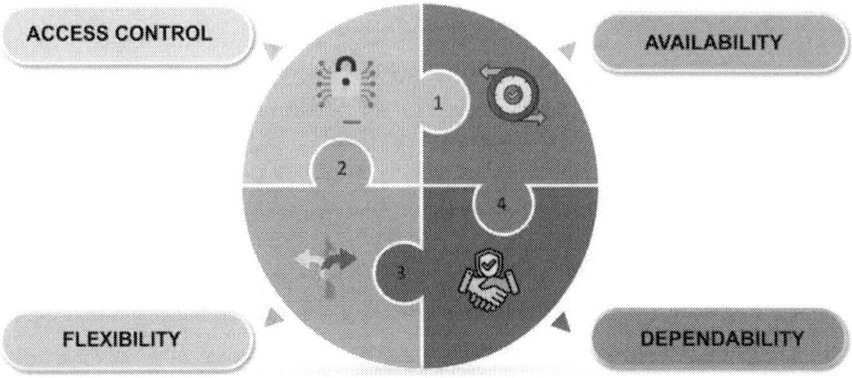

FIGURE 4.6 Security and privacy challenges in healthcare.

verification procedure. The user's identity is verified through authentication before allowing access to data. Moreover, it validates correspondence with a designated person. Based on security policies, the authorization process determines if specific data parts are restricted from external requesters [43]. Additionally, achieving security goals requires a balance between patient availability and confidentiality. It can be achieved through the implementation of an effective access control system.

b. *Availability*: A functional, accessible, and usable system or resource within healthcare system is accessible to authorized users at all times and locations. However, to ensure safe electronic medical care for patients, power outages and device malfunctions should be prevented. Additionally, regular system updates are also crucial for this purpose [44].
c. *Dependability*: Dependability provides complete medical information recovery at all times. However, independent of node loss or network dynamics. Inaccurate data resulting from network issues in medical situations can be fatal and cause significant harm. Additionally, reliability is capacity of a system to tolerate errors, preserving trust by granting reliable and consistent access to vital medical data [45].
d. *Flexibility*: Flexibility is the ability of a healthcare system to modify guidelines governing access to medical records in emergencies. Overly restrictive access to a patient's information can potentially endanger their life. It can also delay their treatment in severe cases. In emergencies, flexibility allows medical staff to quickly access patient data, even when it's not typically permitted [46].

4.6 PRIVACY CONCERNS WITH AI IN HEALTHCARE

AI in healthcare presents significant data protection challenges. It results in the need for strong security solutions to prevent unauthorized access. More interestingly, the

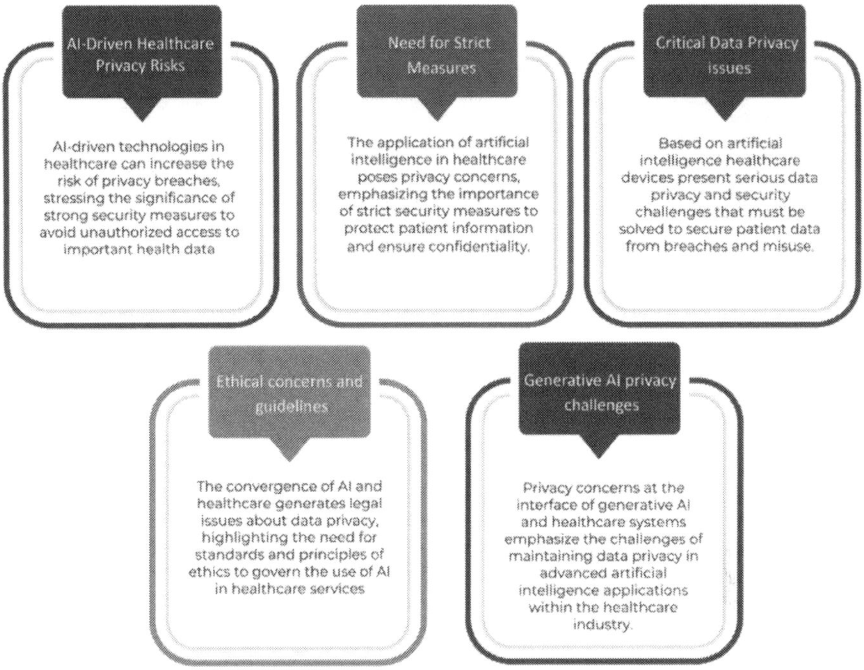
AI-Driven Healthcare Privacy Risks
AI-driven technologies in healthcare can increase the risk of privacy breaches, stressing the significance of strong security measures to avoid unauthorized access to important health data
Need for Strict Measures
The application of artificial intelligence in healthcare poses privacy concerns, emphasizing the importance of strict security measures to protect patient information and ensure confidentiality.
Critical Data Privacy issues
Based on artificial intelligence healthcare devices present serious data privacy and security challenges that must be solved to secure patient data from breaches and misuse.
Ethical concerns and guidelines
The convergence of AI and healthcare generates legal issues about data privacy, highlighting the need for standards and principles of ethics to govern the use of AI in healthcare services
Generative AI privacy challenges
Privacy concerns at the interface of generative AI and healthcare systems emphasize the challenges of maintaining data privacy in advanced artificial intelligence applications within the healthcare industry.

FIGURE 4.7 Privacy issues with AI in healthcare.

integration of AI and healthcare has led to the creation of ethical guidelines and standards to regulate the use of AI in healthcare services. Figure 4.7 illustrates AI privacy issues in healthcare. However, to prevent data breaches, strong security measures are required. Additionally, use of AI in healthcare raises ethical concerns, necessitating development of ethical standards for its application. Moreover, the integration of AI and healthcare systems demonstrates the necessity of robust data protection laws [47].

4.7 DATA PRIVACY AND AI IN HEALTHCARE

Healthcare technology is always evolving; therefore, it's important to take security and data privacy into account while developing AI-based healthcare solutions. Privacy concerns arise because AI in healthcare requires access to personal medical data. However, securing sensitive data and adhering to privacy rules require robust security measures. Figure 4.8 illustrates the use of AI and data privacy in healthcare. Moreover, ethical concerns surrounding data privacy necessitate responsible use of AI technology. Additionally, patient privacy and data protection depend on adherence to legal frameworks such as Health Insurance Probability and Accountability Act (HIPAA) [48].

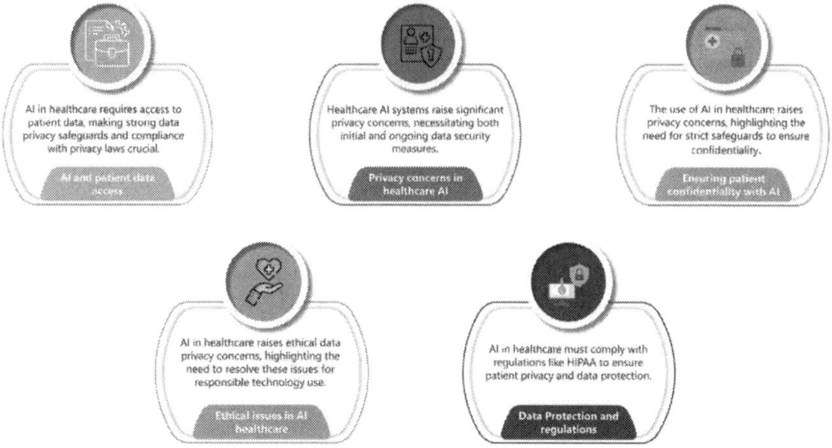

FIGURE 4.8 AI and data privacy in healthcare.

4.8 NEED FOR SECURITY AND PRIVACY STANDARDS

Adoption of AI in healthcare necessitates implementation of robust privacy and security standards to address evolving data privacy and security issues. Figure 4.9 presents requirements for security and privacy standards in healthcare.

i. Developing operational guidelines for AI in healthcare is essential to ensuring patient data protection, promoting informed privacy management, and strengthening privacy legislation [49].
ii. As AI gains prominence in healthcare, security and privacy rules become crucial to protect patient data, mitigate risks, and ensure legal compliance [50].
iii. Implementation of AI in healthcare is dependent upon obtaining patient medical records, underscoring the necessity of enforcing stringent security and privacy protocols. It safeguards confidential information and maintains patient anonymity.
iv. Use of AI in healthcare raises privacy concerns. It needs clear security and privacy guidelines to effectively manage these concerns and maintain patient trust.

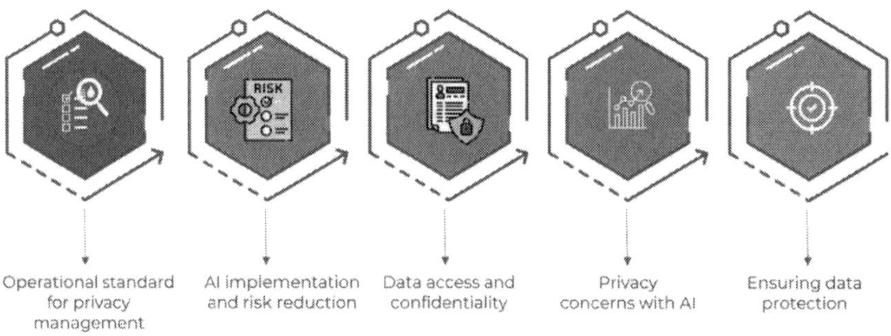

FIGURE 4.9 Need for security and privacy in healthcare.

4.9 IMPROVING HEALTHCARE DATA SECURITY THROUGH AI

AI can improve healthcare data security by preventing security breaches and ensuring data safety. Moreover, it enhances industry's overall data security. A consistent policy for healthcare data security is crucial since effective collaboration among security, AI, and IT departments is essential to preserving data safety in AI era [51].

AI-powered systems are a valuable tool for healthcare organizations to enhance patient data security. It highlights the significance of utilizing AI to effectively protect electronically protected health information. However, ensuring data privacy in healthcare industry, particularly in the age of AI is crucial for protecting patient confidentiality [52]. AI is revolutionizing healthcare industry by improving privacy and security protocols to safeguard patient data. Additionally, the development of healthcare technology necessitates the adoption of AI technologies to enhance data security; however, it is committed to maintaining ethical standards and adherence to privacy laws. Prioritizing security and privacy issues becomes increasingly important as AI develops to preserve sensitive health data and the integrity of healthcare systems [53].

4.10 SECURITY AND PRIVACY REQUIREMENTS FOR HEALTHCARE SYSTEM

Modern healthcare systems face higher security and privacy challenges than other internet-based systems. Security and privacy needs at different levels of healthcare system vary depending on how they function. A detailed examination and discussion of these requirements are presented in Figure 4.10.

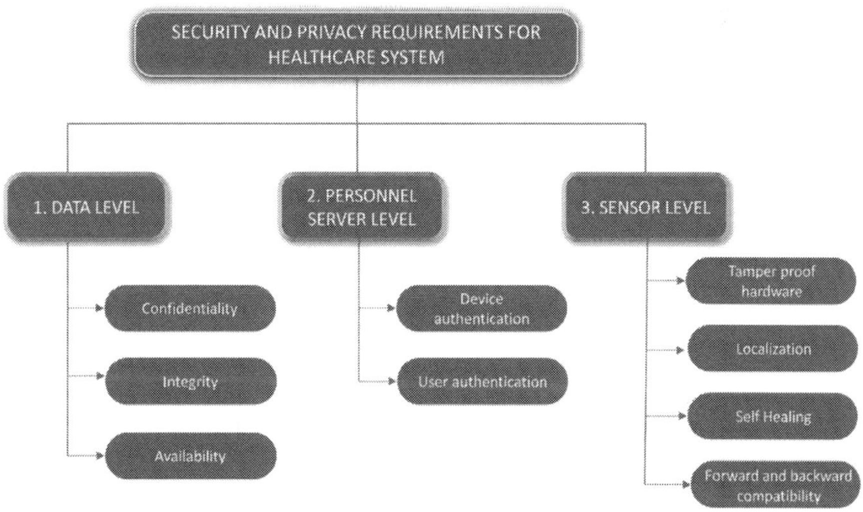

FIGURE 4.10 Security and privacy requirements for healthcare systems.

4.10.1 Data Level

a. *Confidentiality*: Data exchanged between medical professionals and their patients is restricted by privacy regulations. However, consent from patients must always be obtained before sharing medical information with healthcare professionals. HIPAA and General Data Production Regulation (GDPR) are privacy rules that govern the collection and use of patient health data [54]. Moreover, access is granted to those who are authorized. Moreover, to stop incidents, patient health data confidentiality must be upheld. It is crucial to delete patient personal data after processing because it can be sold on black markets by cyber criminals; additionally, with the exception of archival, scientific, historical, or statistical objectives, data should be permanently removed from database [55].

b. *Integrity*: Data integrity is a process of ensuring that information is accurate, efficient, and consistent. In the medical field, it is essential to protect patient privacy, especially regarding diagnostic and laboratory test findings. For researchers and healthcare professionals, maintaining data integrity is a challenging task. Moreover, governments aim to enhance patient care by introducing computerized medical records. Healthcare record computerization is causing great concern among security specialists [56]. However, the frequency of confidentiality attacks, privacy invasions, and data breaches is on the rise. A patient's life could be in danger if medical records are tampered with. Data integrity requirements in healthcare sector ensure that information is transmitted wirelessly and reaches its destination undamaged. Moreover, attackers might change patient data via wireless transfer and put patients in danger. Additionally, implementing appropriate safeguards is crucial to prevent malicious attacks from altering data [57].

c. *Availability*: Healthcare workers require constant access to services and data, necessitating digitization of patient records. DoS attacks have the potential to make vital data gathered from medical servers and devices unavailable. However, device's failure to send timely notifications during a heart attack could potentially lead to fatal situations. Healthcare gadgets and apps should be activated to ensure data access and prevent data loss. Additionally, medical staff should promptly restore patient data to prevent DoS attacks.

4.10.2 Personnel Server Level

Data is usually collected and aggregated by healthcare systems on personal servers and then transferred to medical servers. Personal server security and privacy are achieved through the use of two different authentication procedures. These authentication procedures are device authentication and user authentication [58].

a. *Device Authentication*: Patient data from medical devices and sensors is stored on a personal server, such as a smartphone. Therefore, before accepting input from these sensory devices, they need to offer some kind of validation [59]. However, secure and encrypted connections are required by authentication method to guarantee data integrity and confidentiality. Sensor-based healthcare systems require device authentication to prevent unauthorized devices from altering patient data. It can potentially impact clinical diagnostic and treatment decisions. Mutual authentication is utilized by personal servers and gadgets due to their superior processing capacity and power compared to medical devices and sensors [60].

b. *User Authentication*: Patients and medical professionals must have access to data stored on personal servers, whether it is kept there temporarily or permanently. Therefore, user authentication methods must be robust. However, smart healthcare systems should use personal servers to provide patient data access during emergencies such as strokes. Moreover, personal servers can utilize biometric authentication by collecting data from patients' sensor devices, such as health or medical equipment [61]. E-health services utilize sensors with limited computer power and backup. Additionally, these services are gaining popularity due to people's busy lifestyles. However, sensor data security and privacy are important issues. However, for security reasons, sensor data is usually saved on personal servers. Moreover, a lightweight authentication system with minimal communication overhead is required by security protocols of these sensors.

4.10.3 Sensor Level

Widespread use of e-health services can be attributed to people's hectic lives. These services gather crucial health data by utilizing sensors with limited computational power and power backup. However, privacy and security of sensor data are still major issues. To maintain security of sensor data, it is frequently stored on personal servers. Additionally, sensor security requires a lightweight and cost-effective authentication technique [62, 63].

a. *Tamper-Proof Hardware*: Important healthcare data can be obtained by attackers by use of sensors, especially environmental sensors. To track communications secretly, attackers can reprogram stolen sensors and equipment. However, physically unclonable functions (PUFs) identify and verify devices based on their inherent physical distinctions. It helps in preventing data manipulation from devices and sensors [64].
b. *Localization*: There are two types of sensor localization used by healthcare technologies. This localization includes sensor/patient location and on-body sensor position. It is essential to localize sensors on body to ensure their correct positioning. However, position identification is crucial for applications like activity recognition. Sensor/Patient localization detects patients whether they are inside or outside a building. Sensors and wearables' mobility allows them to move within and outside network's coverage area. Moreover, real-time sensor detection is necessary if network allows regular departure and return of detectors.
c. *Self-healing*: Healthcare wearables and sensors provide self-healing capabilities. It is having the ability to resume functions following incidents

of security [65]. Devices should be capable of recognizing and analysing assaults without human assistance. Additionally, it implements appropriate security measures. These methods need to be low-impact and reduce the overhead of network connections.

d. *Forward and Backward Compatibility*: Forward compatibility is a process of ensuring that medical sensors cannot read messages once they have left network. However, newly connected sensors are unable to properly read messages provided by previous systems due to backward compatibility [66]. Moreover, faulty sensors in healthcare sector need to be changed frequently. Additionally, both forward and backward compatibility are requirements for sensors.

4.11 FUTURE RESEARCH DIRECTIONS

As AI technology plays a bigger role in healthcare, future research must concentrate on improving privacy, security, and ethical norms. To stay current with technological advancements, research should focus on renovating privacy-preserving methods, creating flexible security structures, and modernizing legal frameworks. Secure and ethical adoption of AI in healthcare systems hinges on its seamless integration and public awareness through education. AI healthcare solutions can enhance patient data security and assurance in future.

4.12 CONCLUSION

In conclusion, application of AI in healthcare represents a significant development. However, it still raises privacy and data security concerns. AI systems must be implemented with a thorough approach to their design and protection. Data protection and appropriate security measures are essential for addressing privacy issues. However, organizations must be proactive in enhancing security frameworks and staying updated with technology advancements, particularly as AI continues to evolve. The healthcare sector can optimize AI's benefits while adhering to data protection regulations by implementing advanced security measures and promoting privacy. AI in healthcare security requires advanced security solutions and a privacy culture to ensure data protection and patient care. In the end, this chapter explores the application of AI in healthcare, discussing developments, architectural approaches, security issues, privacy concerns, and ways to enhance data security.

REFERENCES

1. Khan, Muhammad Adnan. "Challenges facing the application of IoT in medicine and healthcare." *International Journal of Computations, Information and Manufacturing (IJCIM)* 1, no. 1 (2021).
2. Vellela, Sai Srinivas, B. Venkateswara Reddy, Kancharla K. Chaitanya, and M. Venkateswara Rao. "An Integrated Approach to Improve e-Healthcare System Using Dynamic Cloud Computing Platform." In *2023 5th International Conference on Smart Systems and Inventive Technology (ICSSIT)*, pp. 776–782. IEEE, 2023.

3. Shi, Shuyun, Debiao He, Li Li, Neeraj Kumar, Muhammad Khurram Khan, and Kim-Kwang Raymond Choo. "Applications of blockchain in ensuring the security and privacy of electronic health record systems: A survey." *Computers & Security* 97 (2020): 101966.
4. Saraswat, Deepti, Pronaya Bhattacharya, Ashwin Verma, Vivek Kumar Prasad, Sudeep Tanwar, Gulshan Sharma, Pitshou N. Bokoro, and Ravi Sharma. "Explainable AI for healthcare 5.0: opportunities and challenges." *IEEE Access* 10 (2022): 84486–84517.
5. Zeadally, Sherali, Farhan Siddiqui, Zubair Baig, and Ahmed Ibrahim. "Smart healthcare: Challenges and potential solutions using internet of things (IoT) and big data analytics." *PSU Research Review* 4, no. 2 (2020): 149–168.
6. Ganiga, Raghavendra, Radhika M. Pai, and Rajesh Kumar Sinha. "Security framework for cloud based electronic health record (EHR) system." *International Journal of Electrical and Computer Engineering* 10, no. 1 (2020): 455.
7. Alabdulatif, Abdulatif, Ibrahim Khalil, and Mohammad Saidur Rahman. "Security of blockchain and AI-empowered smart healthcare: application-based analysis." *Applied Sciences* 12, no. 21 (2022): 11039.
8. Qayyum, Adnan, Junaid Qadir, Muhammad Bilal, and Ala Al-Fuqaha. "Secure and robust machine learning for healthcare: A survey." *IEEE Reviews in Biomedical Engineering* 14 (2020): 156–180.
9. Alshehri, F. and G. Muhammad. "A comprehensive survey of the Internet of Things (IoT) and AI-based smart healthcare." *IEEE Access* 9 (2020): 3660–3678.
10. Ghazal, Taher M. "Internet of things with artificial intelligence for health care security." *Arabian Journal for Science and Engineering* 48, no. 4 (2021): 5689–5689.
11. Zaman, Umar, Imran, Faisal Mehmood, Naeem. Iqbal, Jungsuk Kim, and Muhammad Ibrahim. "Towards secure and intelligent internet of health things: A survey of enabling technologies and applications." *Electronics* 11, no. 12 (2022): 1893.
12. Albahri, Ahmed Shihab, Ali M. Duhaim, Mohammed A. Fadhel, Alhamzah Alnoor, Noor S. Baqer, Laith Alzubaidi, and Osamah Shihab Albahri et al. "A systematic review of trustworthy and explainable artificial intelligence in healthcare: Assessment of quality, bias risk, and data fusion." *Information Fusion* 96 (2023): 156–191.
13. Almalawi, Abdulmohsen, Asif Irshad Khan, Fawaz Alsolami, Yoosef B. Abushark, and Ahmed S. Alfakeeh. "Managing security of healthcare data for a modern healthcare system." *Sensors* 23, no. 7 (2023): 3612.
14. Patil, Sanjay, and Harish Shankar. "Transforming healthcare: harnessing the power of AI in the modern era." *International Journal of Multidisciplinary Sciences and Arts* 2, no. 1 (2023): 60–70.
15 Elnawawy, Mohammed., Hallajiyan, Mohammadreza., Mitra, Gargi., Iqbal, Shahrear., and Pattabiraman, Karthik. (2024). Systematically Assessing the Security Risks of AI/ML-enabled Connected Healthcare Systems. *arXiv preprint arXiv:2401.17136.*
16 Stilinski, Delan and John Owen. (2024). Federated Learning for Secure and Decentralized AI in the Internet of Things (IoT).
17. Keshta, Ismail and Ammar Odeh. "Security and privacy of electronic health records: Concerns and challenges." *Egyptian Informatics Journal* 22, no. 2 (2021): 177–183.
18. Rasheed, Khansa, Adnan Qayyum, Mohammed Ghaly, Ala Al-Fuqaha, Adeel Razi, and Junaid Qadir. "Explainable, trustworthy, and ethical machine learning for healthcare: A survey." *Computers in Biology and Medicine* 149 (2022): 106043.
19. Pradhan, Bikash, Saugat Bhattacharyya, and Kunal Pal. "IoT-based applications in healthcare devices." *Journal of Healthcare Engineering* 2021, no. 1 (2021): 6632599.
20. Suleski, Tance, Mohiuddin Ahmed, Wencheng Yang, and Eugene Wang. "A review of multi-factor authentication in the Internet of Healthcare Things." *Digital Health* 9 (2023), doi:10.1177/20552076231177144

21. Shinde, Rucha, Shruti Patil, Ketan Kotecha, Vidyasagar Potdar, Ganeshsree Selvachandran, and Ajith Abraham. "Securing AI-based healthcare systems using blockchain technology: A state-of-the-art systematic literature review and future research directions." *Transactions on Emerging Telecommunications Technologies* 35, no. 1 (2024): e4884.
22. Sharma, Pratima, Suyel Namasudra, Naveen Chilamkurti, Byung-Gyu Kim, and Ruben Gonzalez Crespo. "Blockchain-based privacy preservation for IoT-enabled healthcare system." *ACM Transactions on Sensor Networks* 19, no. 3 (2023): 1–17.
23. Kuznetsov, Alexandr, Paolo Sernani, Luca Romeo, Emanuele Frontoni, and Adriano Mancini. "On the integration of artificial intelligence and blockchain technology: A perspective about security." *IEEE Access* 12, (2024): 3881–3897.
24. Saha, Sayantani, Chandreyee Chowdhury, and Sarmistha Neogy. "A novel two phase data sensitivity based access control framework for healthcare data." *Multimedia Tools and Applications* 83, no. 3 (2024): 8867–8892.
25. Mennella, Ciro, Umberto Maniscalco, Giuseppe De Pietro, and Massimo Esposito. "Ethical and regulatory challenges of AI technologies in healthcare: A narrative review." *Heliyon*, 10, no. 4 (2024).
26. Arigbabu, Aisha Temitope, Oluwaseun Oladeji Olaniyi, Chinasa Susan Adigwe, Olubukola Omolara Adebiyi, and Samson Abidemi Ajayi. "Data governance in AI-enabled healthcare systems: A case of the project nightingale." *Asian Journal of Research in Computer Science* 17, no. 5 (2024): 85–107.
27. Mazumder, Md Samiul Alam. "The Transformative Impact of Big Data in Healthcare: Improving Outcomes, Safety, and Efficiencies." *Global Mainstream Journal of Business, Economics, Development & Project Management* 3, no. 03 (2024): 01–12.
28. Hick, John L., Eric S. Toner, Dan Hanfling, Paul D. Biddinger, and James V. Lawler. "Data and disasters: Essential information needed for all healthcare threats." *Health Security* 22, no. 1 (2024): 3–10.
29. Alhur, Anas. "Redefining healthcare with artificial intelligence (AI): The contributions of ChatGPT, Gemini, and Co-pilot." *Cureus* 16, no. 4 (2024).
30. Vatambeti, Ramesh, ES Phalguna Krishna, M. Ganesh Karthik, and Vijay Kumar Damera. "Securing the medical data using enhanced privacy preserving based blockchain technology in Internet of Things." *Cluster Computing* 27, no. 2 (2024): 1625–1637.
31. Adeghe, Ehizogie Paul, Chioma Anthonia Okolo, and Olumuyiwa Tolulope Ojeyinka. "A review of emerging trends in telemedicine: Healthcare delivery transformations." *International Journal of Life Science Research Archive* 6, no. 1 (2024): 137–147.
32. Oyeniyi, Johnson. "The role of AI and mobile apps in patient-centric healthcare delivery." *World Journal of Advanced Research and Reviews* 22, no. 1 (2024): 1897–1907.
33. Ibeh, Chidera Victoria, Oluwafunmi Adijat Elufioye, Temidayo Olorunsogo, Onyeka Franca Asuzu, Ndubuisi Leonard Nduubuisi, and Andrew Ifesinachi Daraojimba. "Data analytics in healthcare: A review of patient-centric approaches and healthcare delivery." *World Journal of Advanced Research and Reviews* 21, no. 2 (2024): 1750–1760.
34. Udegbe, Francisca Chibugo, Ogochukwu Roseline Ebulue, Charles Chukwudalu Ebulue, and Chukwunonso Sylvester Ekesiobi. "The role of artificial intelligence in healthcare: A systematic review of applications and challenges." *International Medical Science Research Journal* 4, no. 4 (2024): 500–508.
35. Abdugapparovna, Mamasolieva Shoxis, and Karimov Abduxalim Abdurazzaqovich. "The need to ensure economic security in the health sector." *Web of Medicine: Journal of Medicine, Practice and Nursing* 2, no. 1 (2024): 75–78.
36. Atadoga, Akoh, Toritsemogba Tosanbami Omaghomi, Oluwafunmi Adijat Elufioye, Ifeoma Pamela Odilibe, Andrew Ifesinachi Daraojimba, and Oluwaseyi Rita Owolabi. "Internet of Things (IoT) in healthcare: A systematic review of use cases and benefits." *International Journal of Science and Research Archive* 11, no. 1 (2024): 1511–1517.

37. Settipalli, Lavanya, G. R. Gangadharan, and Sivaiah Bellamkonda. "An extended lightweight blockchain based collaborative healthcare system for fraud prevention." *Cluster Computing* 27, no. 1 (2024): 563–573.
38. Ahad, Abdul, Zheng Jiangbina, Mohammad Tahir, Ibraheem Shayea, Muhammad Aman Sheikh, and Faizan Rasheed. "6G and Intelligent Healthcare: Taxonomy, technologies, open issues and future research directions." *Internet of Things*, *25* (2024): 101068.
39. Kuliha, Megha, and Sunita Verma. "Secure internet of medical things based electronic health records scheme in trust decentralized loop federated learning consensus blockchain." *International Journal of Intelligent Networks* 5 (2024): 161–174.
40. Wells, Alec, and Aminu Bello Usman. "Privacy and biometrics for smart healthcare systems: Attacks, and techniques." *Information Security Journal: A Global Perspective* 33, no. 3 (2024): 307–331.
41. Alghamdi, Ahmed Mohammed, Mahmoud Ahmad Al-Khasawneh, Ala Alarood, and Eesa Alsolami. "The role of machine learning in managing and organizing healthcare records." *Engineering, Technology & Applied Science Research* 14, no. 2 (2024): 13695–13701.
42. Eswaran, Ushaa., and Alex Khang. (2024). Artificial Intelligence (AI)-Aided Computer Vision (CV) in Healthcare System. In *Computer Vision and AI-Integrated IoT Technologies in the Medical Ecosystem* (pp. 125–137). CRC Press.
43. Puri, Vikram, Aman Kataria, and Vishal Sharma. "Artificial intelligence-powered decentralized framework for Internet of Things in Healthcare 4.0." *Transactions on Emerging Telecommunications Technologies* 35, no. 4 (2024): e4245.
44. Singh, Puneet. "Transforming Healthcare through AI: Enhancing Patient Outcomes and Bridging Accessibility Gaps." *Journal of Artificial Intelligence Research* 4, no. 1 (2024): 220–232.
45. Malathi, J, K. R. Kusha, Samson. Isaac, Alabazar. Ramesh, M. Rajendiran, and Sampath Boopathi. (2024). IoT-Enabled Remote Patient Monitoring for Chronic Disease Management and Cost Savings: Transforming Healthcare. In *Advances in Explainable AI Applications for Smart Cities* (pp. 371–388). IGI Global.
46. Singh, G., D. Tiwari, P. Goel, P. Vishwakarma, K. Gupta, and A. Verma. "Cybersecurity Challenges In Healthcare Systems." *2024 International Conference on Communication, Computer Sciences and Engineering (IC3SE)*, Gautam Buddha Nagar, India, 2024, pp. 1–6, doi: 10.1109/IC3SE62002.2024.10593022
47. Gupta, Arnav. and Sujata. Joshi. "Emerging Trends and Scope of Healthcare Analytics." *2022 International Interdisciplinary Humanitarian Conference for Sustainability (IIHC)*, Bengaluru, India, 2022, pp. 93–101, doi: 10.1109/IIHC55949.2022.10059883
48. Sharif, Muhammad. Irfan., Jian. Ping. Li, Sana. Ullah, Amin. Ul Haq, and Gulzar. Alam. "An Efficient Access Privacy Protocol for Healthcare Patient Information System." *2019 16th International Computer Conference on Wavelet Active Media Technology and Information Processing*, Chengdu, China, 2019, pp. 461–465, doi: 10.1109/ICCWAMTIP47768.2019.9067602
49. Verma, P. and A. K. Jain. "A Comprehensive Study on the Application of Blockchain Technology's Use in Healthcare." *2023 International Conference on Sustainable Computing and Smart Systems (ICSCSS)*, Coimbatore, India, 2023, pp. 1388–1393, doi: 10.1109/ICSCSS57650.2023.10169250
50. Awotunde, Joseph. Bamidele., Sakinat. Oluwabukonla. Folorunso, Sunday. Adeola. Ajagbe, Jatinder. Garg, and Gbemisola. Janet Ajamu. (2022). AiIoMT: IoMT-based system-enabled artificial intelligence for enhanced smart healthcare systems. In Machine Learning for Critical Internet of Medical Things: Applications and Use Cases (pp. 229–254), Springer Nature.

51. KumarChaudhary, Ravi. Raushan., Kakali. Chatterjee, and Ashish. Singh. "A Health Monitoring Framework Based on Edge of Things for Smart Healthcare System." *2021 IEEE 6th International Conference on Computing, Communication and Automation (ICCCA)*, Arad, Romania, 2021, pp. 339–344, doi: 10.1109/ICCCA52192.2021.9666367
52. Ajibade, Samuel-Soma., Angla. Siew. Hoong. Lee, Muhammed. Basheer. Jasser, and Tomiwa. Faith. Akinola. "Application of Artificial Intelligence in Healthcare Systems: A Scientometric Analysis." *2024 International Conference on Science, Engineering and Business for Driving Sustainable Development Goals (SEB4SDG)*, Omu-Aran, Nigeria, 2024, pp. 1–5, doi: 10.1109/SEB4SDG60871.2024.10630087
53. Mana, Suja Cherukullapurath., G. Kalaiarasi, L. Suji. Helen, and R. Senthamil Selvi. "Application of Machine Learning in Healthcare: An Analysis." *2022 3rd International Conference on Electronics and Sustainable Communication Systems (ICESC)*, Coimbatore, India, 2022, pp. 1611–1615, doi: 10.1109/ICESC54411.2022.9885296
54. Al-Anezi, Fahad. M., Sharifah. Alrajhi, Nouf. M. Al-Anezi, Dhabia. Mohammad. Alabbadi, and Rayna. Almana. "A review of healthcare system in Saudi Arabia." *2020 19th International Symposium on Distributed Computing and Applications for Business Engineering and Science (DCABES)*, Xuzhou, China, 2020, pp. 318–322, doi: 10.1109/DCABES50732.2020.00088
55. Ramar, Kaladevi., Gopirajan. P. V, Hariharan. Shanmugasundaram, Bhanu. Prasad. Andraju, and Sandhiya. Baskar. "Digital Healthcare using Blockchain." *2022 1st International Conference on Computational Science and Technology (ICCST)*, CHENNAI, India, 2022, pp. 651–655, doi: 10.1109/ICCST55948.2022.10040411
56. Jameil, Ahmed. K. and Hamed. Al-Raweshidy. "AI-Enabled Healthcare and Enhanced Computational Resource Management with Digital Twins Into Task Offloading Strategies." *IEEE Access* 12 (2024): 90353–90370. doi: 10.1109/ACCESS.2024.3420741
57. Adwer, Lina. and Erik. Whiting. "Exploring Artificial Intelligence Solutions and Challenges in Healthcare Administration." *2024 IEEE 12th International Conference on Healthcare Informatics (ICHI)*, Orlando, FL, USA, 2024, pp. 528–530, doi: 10.1109/ICHI61247.2024.00077
58. Naidu, P. Ramesh., Dankan. Gowda, Parismita. Sarma, Dinesh. Arora, Sampathirao. Suneetha, and Sandip. Ramesh. Patil. "Advancements in Multi-Cloud Applications for Enhanced E-Healthcare Services," *2023 International Conference on Artificial Intelligence for Innovations in Healthcare Industries (ICAIIHI)*, Raipur, India, 2023, pp. 1–7, doi: 10.1109/ICAIIHI57871.2023.10488961
59. Al-Jaroodi, Jameela., Nader. Mohamed, N. Kesserwan, and Imad. Jawhar. "Healthcare 4.0 – Managing a Holistic Transformation." *2022 IEEE International Systems Conference (SysCon)*, Montreal, QC, Canada, 2022, pp. 1–8, doi: 10.1109/SysCon53536.2022.9773863
60. Mistry, Jimit.; & Natalia. M. Arzeno. "Document Understanding for Healthcare Referrals," *2023 IEEE 11th International Conference on Healthcare Informatics (ICHI)*, Houston, TX, USA, 2023, pp. 160–161, doi: 10.1109/ICHI57859.2023.00067
61. Demirkan, Haluk. "A Smart Healthcare Systems Framework." *IT Professional* 15, no. 5 (Sept.-Oct. 2013): 38–45. doi: 10.1109/MITP.2013.35
62. Zhu, Hongxu. *et al.* "Smart Healthcare in the Era of Internet-of-Things." *IEEE Consumer Electronics Magazine* 8, no. 5 (Sept. 2019): pp. 26–30. doi: 10.1109/MCE.2019.2923929
63. Bt Nasaruddin, Nurul. Shazmin., Izzatdin. Abdul. Aziz, and Noor. Adilah. Rashid. "Web-Based Electronic Healthcare Record System (EHRS) Based on Feedback." *2018 IEEE Conference on Application, Information and Network Security (AINS)*, Langkawi, Malaysia, 2018, pp. 27–32, doi: 10.1109/AINS.2018.8631427.

64. Tania, Marzia. Hoque.; & David. A. Clifton. "Unleashing the Power of Federated Learning in Fragmented Digital Healthcare Systems: A Visionary Perspective." *2023 15th International Conference on Software, Knowledge, Information Management and Applications (SKIMA)*, Kuala Lumpur, Malaysia, 2023, pp. 40–44, doi: 10.1109/SKIMA59232.2023.10387304.
65. Sermontyte-Baniule, Rima. and Asta. Pundziene. "Value-Capture Capabilities in Value-Based Digital Healthcare Performance," *2021 IEEE International Conference on Technology and Entrepreneurship (ICTE)*, Kaunas, Lithuania, 2021, pp. 1–7, doi: 10.1109/ICTE51655.2021.9584684
66. Ramos, Carolina. Castellanos., Angle. Pinto. Mangones, Yair. Rivera. Julio, Juan. Torres. Tovio, Horderlin. Robles. Vega, and Nelson. A. Perez. García. "Leveraging Electronic Healthcare Records Based on ISO/EN 13606 for Enhanced Telemedicine in Rural Colombia," *2023 IEEE Colombian Caribbean Conference (C3)*, Barranquilla, Colombia, 2023, pp. 1–6, doi: 10.1109/C358072.2023.10436243

5 Ensuring Patient-Centric Data Control Using Blockchain in Smart Healthcare System

Manoj Kumar, Urmila Pilania, and Mazdak Zamani

5.1 INTRODUCTION

The traditional healthcare system is transforming into smart healthcare due to blockchain integration. With blockchain healthcare data can be managed, shared, and utilized in well-organized ways [1]. Blockchain can address issues like data security, transparency, reliability, scalability, interoperability, and other inefficiency [2]. Blockchain is immutable and decentralized, because of that it can enhance data security and reliability. All the transactions are recorded on a public ledger and these transactions are accessible to everyone on the network. A transaction once completed cannot be modified resulting in history proof. All the transactions are secured using cryptography algorithms and hashing. Blockchain automates the processes using smart contracts. Smart contracts are the self-executing codes [3].

The blocks are connected using cryptographic hashes resulting in high security of data in blockchain [4]. All the blocks have strong and secure connections. There is no limit on the number of blocks in the blockchain. The blocks are connected and carry information about their neighbor block in the form of a hash [5]. The contributors in blockchain are connected in a peer-to-peer network [6]. Each block has two keys associated with it, one is the public key and another one is the private key. The public key encrypts the message and the private key is used to decode the message [7].

In this work, blockchain architecture is designed for hospitals as shown in Figure 5.1. Smart contracts are created for the management of interactions between entities like patients, doctors, laboratories, and pharmacy. The patient is the first entity that uses smart contracts for login at the site of the hospital. The prescriptions uploaded by the doctors are accessible to the patient and he/she can set access rights for the others. After approval from the patient for adding transactions on the blockchain, it can be added to the blockchain. The review of patient requests, record checking, decision-making, and editing of reports are handled by the second entity of the application which is the doctor. The next entity is the laboratory, which utilizes smart contracts for getting access to patient's prescriptions and uploading the reports generated by the lab followed by payment of bills for the reports. The last entity

 DOI: 10.1201/9781003510932-5

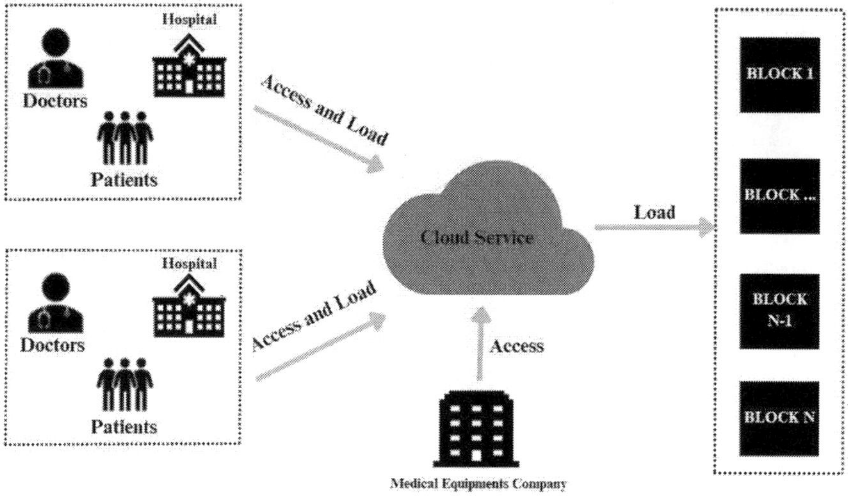

FIGURE 5.1 Proposed blockchain architecture.

used in the work is a pharmacy that gets prescriptions, allots medication, and bills patients/insurance by using smart contracts. The work utilizes smart contracts through blockchain to automate the process and maintain the integrity of the data.

5.2 LITERATURE REVIEW

These days' medical services are a necessary part of everyone's life. IoT with blockchain is playing an important role in everyone's life. In the last five years, measured growth in IoT devices has been observed. Remote patient monitoring is very common in the healthcare sector due to the use of IoT devices. Authors in this work proposed a blockchain-based healthcare system to manage and facilitate patients. The author resolved the issue of high cost and computational power by using blockchain and IoT devices. The proposed model is distributed in nature due to the facility provided by blockchain. Blockchain enhances the security of healthcare data and IoT helps in the collection of data remotely [8]. Blockchain and IoT devices have its applications in many sectors such as medicine, education, industry, and banking. The healthcare industry is growing well because of the integration of IoT and blockchain. The use of blockchain avoids different types of attacks on healthcare data. These attacks may include scaling, collision, phishing, and translation. Sharma et al. [9] proposed a distributed contract-based blockchain system using the Etherscan tool. This tool has been used to calculate computational cost, time, and bandwidth used. The proposed work was also compared with the existing work for computational time, latency, cost, and bandwidth. The proposed work was found to be satisfactory in terms of the mentioned parameters.

Technology is growing day by day and due to this many things are becoming simple for the new generation. These technologies help in the growth of cities to smart cities. Kamruzzaman et al. [10] proposed IoT, blockchain, and fog computing for the innovation of smart cities. They also did a literature review of many papers in the field. The authors of this paper have taken most of the information from PRISMA and AMSTAR. IoT was found to be the most widely used technique and blockchain helps in enhancing the security of patient data. The computational cost and interoperability were also observed as the main issues due to the integration of IoT and blockchain in healthcare. These days due to the involvement of IoT and blockchain healthcare data is maintained electronically by professionals. Maintaining health data electronically helps professionals and patients access data remotely. The increased use of IoT devices is creating problems of security. Mohammed et al. [11] proposed the integration of IoT devices and blockchain using the Django framework. The problem of remote data collection is handled by IoT devices and blockchain provides security to the collected data.

The proposed work [12] was the framework of four layers IoT enabled healthcare data monitoring. It collects data using IoT wearable devices and blockchain applies security to the collected and stored data. Blockchain reduces overload on the network by providing lightweight decentralized architecture. The proposed routing techniques utilize parameters such as probability, reliability, and node energy for the transfer of data. It decreases the load on the network and saves energy. The patient healthcare data was collected using four pre-trained models: ResNet50, VGG19, InceptionV3, and SqueezeNet. For the evaluation of the research work, accuracy has been calculated and it was found to be 92.24%. In work [13], ElRahman and Alluhaidan proposed an IoT-blockchain technique to maintain the integrity of healthcare data. During communication healthcare data goes through different nodes or servers, so there are chances of data modification. The proposed work was found to be user friendly and the integrity of data during communication was also maintained by the authors. It was also compared with other work in the same field.

5.3 PREREQUISITE FOR PROPOSED WORK

The traditional healthcare system has serious issues of data security and privacy. Blockchain is immutable and decentralized, because of that it can enhance data security and reliability [14]. All the transactions are recorded on a public ledger and these transactions are accessible to everyone on the network. A transaction once completed cannot be modified resulting in history proof. All the transactions are secured using cryptography algorithms and hashing [15]. Blockchain automates the processes using smart contracts. Smart contracts are self-executing codes. The sensitive healthcare data is secure by blockchain as central databases are replaced by decentralized approaches. Blockchain networks use smart contracts to systematize healthcare-related tasks like management of patient reports, records of insurance claims, and medical billing.

Blockchain permits smooth data sharing among hospitals, clinics, and research institutes [16]. A single source of information can be efficiently utilized by many organizations because of the capabilities of blockchain. Whenever some tourists visit an emergency hospital, doctors can access the data of patients by using the blockchain-based system, resulting in improved accuracy of diagnosis and treatment along with more care of patients [17]. The transparency feature of blockchain provides the authentication for the validity of medicine at each stage of the supply chain starting from the producer to the patient [18].

The research work is useful for patients, doctors, laboratories, and pharmacies. By using this interface patient data can be organized in a well manner with transparency and safety of data. It provides a unique ID to each patient and patients use this ID for any type of communication through the application. The designed application provides integrity of data, transparency, and detail of data retrieval and updating. The access rights are preserved through smart contracts at various levels. Before any type of action is taken by any of the entities in the application, it asks for permission. The patient is the entity who has access to all the resources available on the application. The application keeps a record of all the transactions like consent of the patient, doctor's prescriptions, medications provided by doctors, and treatment plans. The data stored on the application can be shared further for research purposes among researchers and academicians. The implementation of the work technology required is ReactJS for the front end, Solidity for backend contracts, and Ethereum for blockchain. Hardware requirements are laptop/desktop/mobile, internet connection, minimum 4GB RAM, and minimum 10 GB ROM. Software requirements are the latest web browser, blockchain knowledge, wallet, etc.

Figure 5.2 explains the connections between a smart contract and various entities in the healthcare system for the proposed work. The smart contract is the function

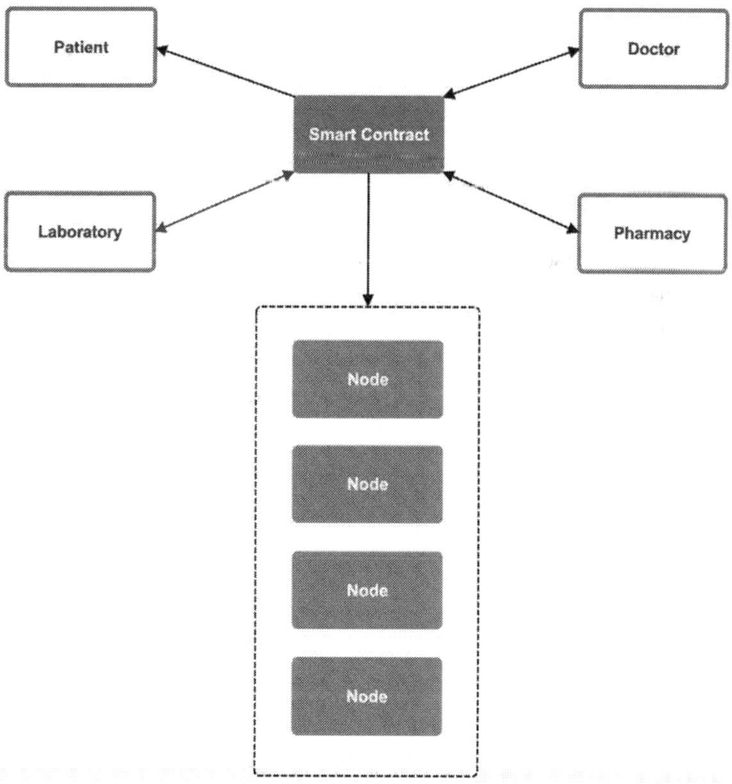

FIGURE 5.2 Architecture design.

that handles the complete application. These are utilized for communication among different entities like patients, doctors, laboratory, and pharmacy

Figure 5.3 describes how different entities in a healthcare system use smart contracts and blockchain to communicate with one another. The figure represents in sequence how users register, how physicians update records, how pharmacists update records, how patients seek medical records, and how laboratories update records. The smart contract makes transparent and safe information sharing among different entities. The records are stored on the blockchain, which ensures security and immutability. The figure represents how to manage healthcare data in a decentralized, safe manner that can improve efficiency and patient privacy.

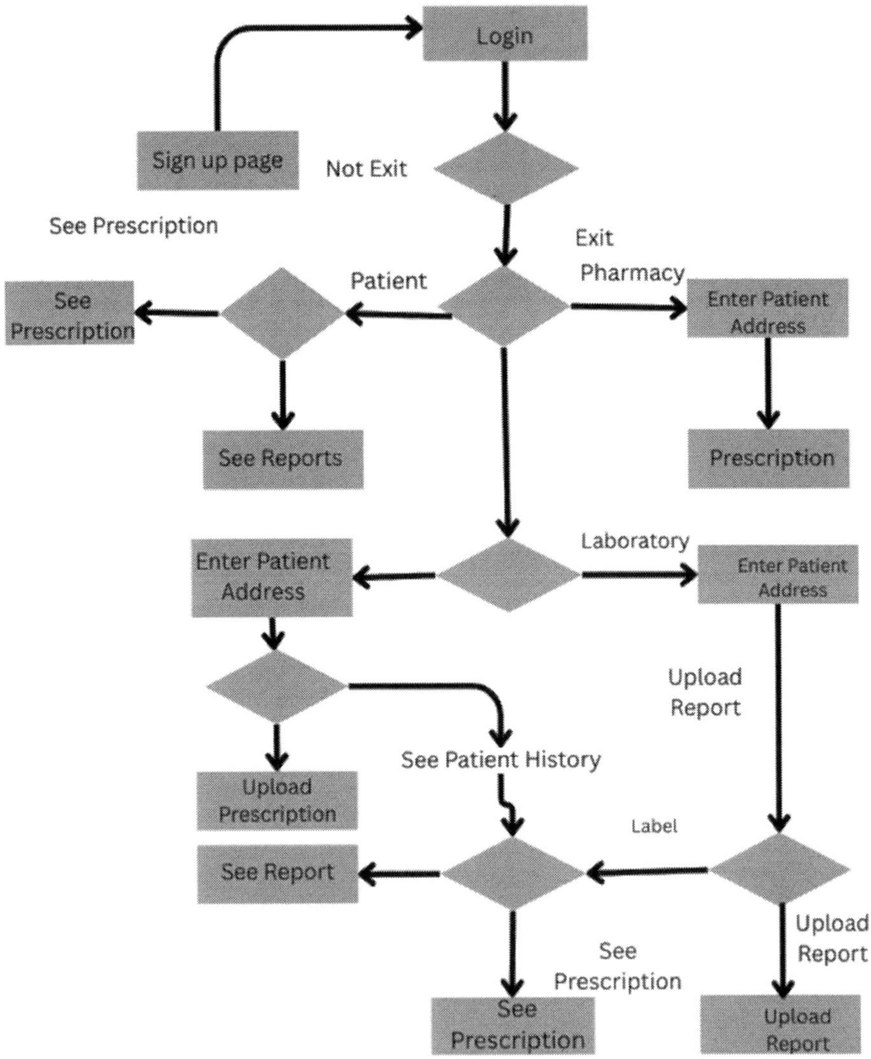

FIGURE 5.3 Flow of data.

In the work user, prescription, doctor, laboratory, and pharmacy represent smart healthcare management. All the relevant information about the entities is stored in the user table. Relevant information may include patient name, doctor name, prescription; timestamp, account detail, etc. are included in the prescription table.

Such files are also maintained in laboratory records and pharmacy records. For fetching the details of patient and doctor from the database, many ways can be utilized. The flow of data is managed through smart contracts. Smart contracts are created for each entity like patient, doctor, pharmacy, and laboratory. Patients log in to the application and access all the records like prescriptions and reports. The smart contract then provides this information to the patient. Subsequently, the patient asks the doctor for their reports and prescriptions. The doctor accesses the blockchain to obtain these documents and sends them to the patient. The patient shares the prescription with the pharmacy, which requests the reports from the laboratory. The laboratory retrieves the reports from the blockchain and sends them to the pharmacy. Finally, the pharmacy sends a report back to the patient. This workflow ensures secure and transparent data sharing among all healthcare participants.

5.4 RESULT AND DISCUSSION

Smart contracts are built on the Ethereum blockchain. Ethereum is the standard platform for the generation of decentralized applications. Smart contracts built on Ethereum are the processes for the automation of complex tasks. These smart contracts reduce the chances of fraud. The decentralized nature of Ethereum guarantees the delivery of data without failure. All the transactions on Ethereum are transparent. Figure 5.4 represents the key features of the proposed work. For the implementation of work, Web3 library import is a must for interaction. JSON ABI (Application Binary Interface) and the address of the login contract are also compulsory. Metamask extension is verified by the loadWeb3 function. If it is present then a Web3 instance with window.ethereum acts as the provider and requests access to the user's Ethereum accounts.

Figure 5.4 represents the key features of the proposed work. React application is utilized to manage client-side routing. It imports various components from different directories, such as home, signup, laboratory, pharmacy, doctor, DoctorLab, DoctorPre, patient, and PatientLab. The loadAccounts function retrieves the user's accounts and authentication status from the blockchain. Patients sign up themselves on the interface for consulting doctors. Doctors can add prescriptions by clicking the "Add Report" button. After the addition of the prescription, it is authenticated by the patient before it is added to the blockchain. If the patient does not authenticate the prescription, then it is not added to the blockchain. On authentication from the patient, it is added to the blockchain and the prescription can be retrieved using the getPatient function. Figure 5.5 represents how to get a report of patient prescriptions.

Clicking on the "Get Report" button, the getPatientReport function is raised. The getPatientReport function checks the patient address field. If the address field is valid

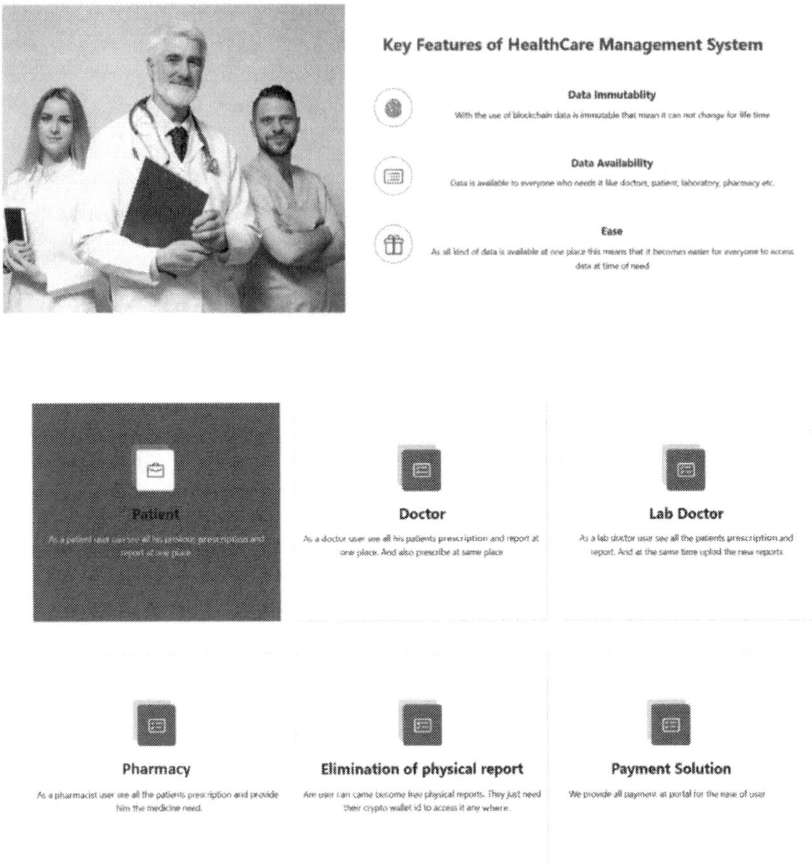

FIGURE 5.4 Key features of proposed work.

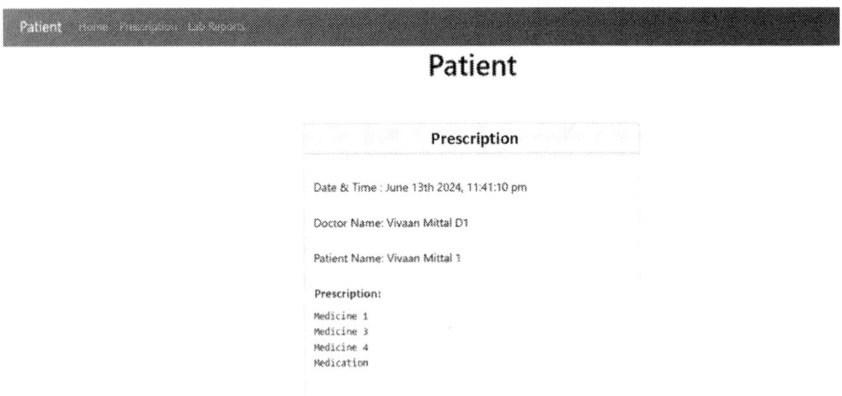

FIGURE 5.5 Patient prescription.

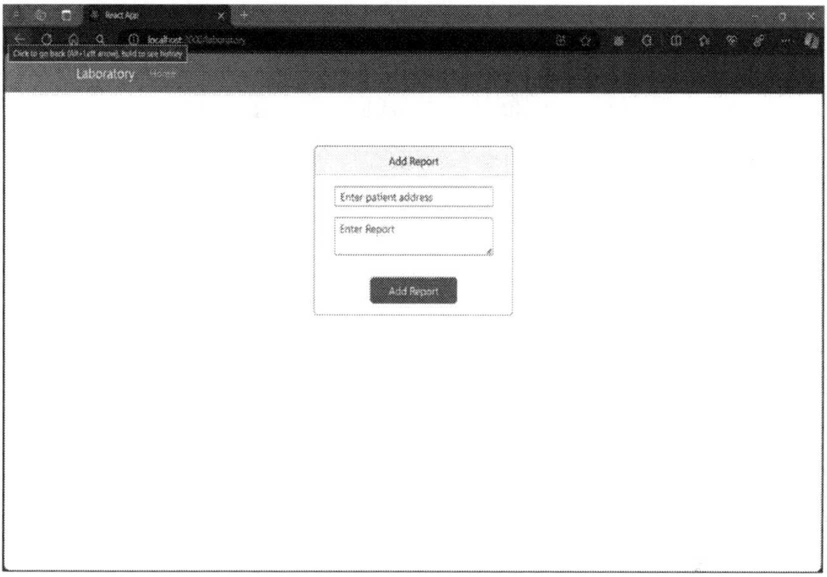

FIGURE 5.6 Patient lab report.

then the getLabReport function is invoked for the authentication from the doctor for adding it to the blockchain. Figure 5.6 shows how to get the patient lab report.

The LabReportCard function is invoked for displaying information on lab reports. Figure 5.7 shows the access to patient reports by the pharmacy. Upon accessing the patient report, the pharmacy provides the required medicine to the patient.

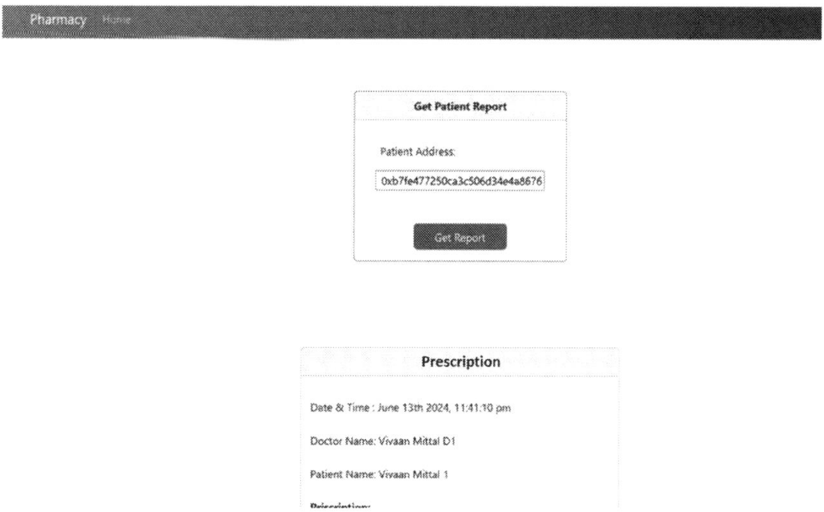

FIGURE 5.7 Patient report access to pharmacy.

The patient has to pay the bill either by insurance or in some other way. The complete process is implemented on the blockchain. Blockchain ensures the security of patient data at various steps by setting authentication mechanisms for patients and doctors. Key issues like integrity of health data, confidentiality, interoperability issues, scalability, and many more issues are handled by the proposed work.

5.5 CONCLUSION

The research work has the potential to transform the way healthcare data is managed, shared, and protected. Through the implementation of blockchain, key challenges are addressed like data security, consistency, integrity, and transparency. The work emphasizes the importance of empowering patients to take control of their health information and participate actively in their care journey. By providing patients with secure digital identities and permission access controls, research work has enabled them to securely access, manage, and share their medical records.

The research work will be overcoming multiple problems in healthcare data management but for the work crypto Ethereum wallet is required. The users who want to use this research work must have a crypto wallet. Having a crypto wallet is not a problem in the city but is a major drawback for villages. Gas fee needs to be submitted every time by a doctor and laboratory to upload prescriptions and reports which may not be liked by many users.

REFERENCES

1. Zaabar, B., Cheikhrouhou, O., Jamil, F., Ammi, M., & Abid, M. (2021). HealthBlock: A secure blockchain-based healthcare data management system. *Computer Networks, 200*, 108500.
2. Khatoon, A. (2020). A blockchain-based smart contract system for healthcare management. *Electronics, 9*(1), 94.
3. Wenzheng, L., Tappaskhanova, M. A., Nikiporets-Takigawa, G., Gorokhova, A. E., & Goncharov, V. V. (2020). Healthcare management: Prospects and risks of using blockchain technology. *Helix-The Scientific Explorer| Peer Reviewed Bimonthly International Journal, 10*(05), 230–235.
4. Bittins, S., Kober, G., Margheri, A., Masi, M., Miladi, A., & Sassone, V. (2021). Healthcare data management by using blockchain technology. Applications of Blockchain in Healthcare (pp. 1–27). Singapore: Springer.
5. Wehbe, Y., Al Zaabi, M., & Svetinovic, D. (2018, November). Blockchain AI Framework for Healthcare Records Management: Constrained Goal Model. In *2018 26th Telecommunications Forum (TELFOR)* (pp. 420–425). IEEE.
6. Pilania, U., Upadhyay, P., Tanwar, R., & Kumar, M. (2023). A Creative Domain of Blockchain Application: NFTs. In *Mobile Radio Communications and 5G Networks: Proceedings of Third MRCN 2022* (pp. 397–406). Singapore: Springer Nature.
7. Pilania, U., Kumar, M., Singh, S., Adhalkha, P., & Satija, T. (2023, December). Securing Confidential Information on WhatsApp with Blockchain Technology. In *International Conference on Advancements in Smart Computing and Information Security* (pp. 53–61). Cham: Springer Nature Switzerland.
8. Dwivedi, A. D., Srivastava, G., Dhar, S., & Singh, R. (2019). A decentralized privacy-preserving healthcare blockchain for IoT. *Sensors, 19*(2), 326.

9. Sharma, P., Namasudra, S., Chilamkurti, N., Kim, B. G., & Gonzalez Crespo, R. (2023). Blockchain-based privacy preservation for IoT-enabled healthcare system. *ACM Transactions on Sensor Networks, 19*(3), 1–17.
10. Kamruzzaman, M. M., Yan, B., Sarker, M. N. I., Alruwaili, O., Wu, M., & Alrashdi, I. (2022). Blockchain and fog computing in IoT-driven healthcare services for smart cities. *Journal of Healthcare Engineering, 2022*(1), 9957888.
11. Mohammed, R., Alubady, R., & Sherbaz, A. (2021, March). Utilizing blockchain technology for IoT-based healthcare systems. In *Journal of Physics: Conference Series* (Vol. 1818, No. 1, p. 012111). IOP Publishing.
12. Rani, P., Kaur, P., Jain, V., Shokeen, J., & Nain, S. (2022). Blockchain-based IoT enabled health monitoring system. *The Journal of Supercomputing, 78*(15), 17284–17308.
13. ElRahman, S. A., & Alluhaidan, A. S. (2021). Blockchain technology and IoT-edge framework for sharing healthcare services. *Soft Computing, 25*(21), 13753–13777.
14. Deepa, N., Devi, T., Gayathri, N., & Kumar, S. R. (2022). Decentralized healthcare management system using blockchain to secure sensitive medical data for users. Blockchain Security in Cloud Computing (pp. 265–282). Springer Nature.
15. Mondal, S., Shafi, M., Gupta, S., & Gupta, S. K. (2022). Blockchain-based secure architecture for electronic healthcare record management. *GMSARN International Journal, 16*(4), 413–26.
16. Jabbar, R., Fetais, N., Krichen, M., & Barkaoui, K. (2020, February). Blockchain technology for healthcare: Enhancing shared electronic health record interoperability and integrity. In *2020 IEEE International Conference on Informatics, IoT, and Enabling Technologies (ICIoT)* (pp. 310–317). IEEE.
17. Vyas, J. D., Han, M., Li, L., Pouriyeh, S., & He, J. S. (2020, April). Integrating blockchain technology into healthcare. In *Proceedings of the 2020 ACM Southeast Conference* (pp. 197–203).
18. Khan, A. I., ALGhamdi, A. S. A. M., Alsolami, F. J., Abushark, Y. B., Almalawi, A., Ali, A. M., ... & Khan, R. A. (2022). Integrating blockchain technology into healthcare through an intelligent computing technique. *Computers, Materials & Continua, 70*(2), 2835–2860.

6 Interface for Monitoring and Tracking Pregnant Women's Fetal Health Conditions Based on Cardiotocogram Information

Aniket Kumar, Manish Kumar, R. Girija, Shefali Singhal, and Shilpi Gupta

6.1 INTRODUCTION

In the medical industry, tracking fetal growth throughout pregnancy is one of the trickiest and most complex procedures. The World Health Organization (WHO) reports that, despite the implementation of preventive measures, approximately 810 pregnant women still pass away every day. In affluent nations, the maternal mortality ratio (MMR) is significantly lower than in developing nations. Typical issues underlying high MMR include maternal diabetes, pre-eclampsia, and inadequate monitoring of the mother's and unborn child's health. With the right medical attention, MMR can be decreased and avoided. Fetal monitoring is a routine technique performed in the third trimester. Fetal monitoring involves assessing the unborn child's health. The health of the mother has a direct impact on fetal growth. Cardiotocography (CTG) is used to continuously measure the health and growth rate of the fetus in order to prevent such issues. The goal of the CTG is to assess the mother's uterine contractions (UC) while simultaneously monitoring the fetus's heartbeat. This procedure would be carried out in the last trimester, after the fetus's development and heart rate are fully integrated. Since this approach is simple and thought to be cost-effective, medical professionals should use it to diagnose fetal status early and lower fetal mortality. CTG results will show the mother's UC and, most significantly, the fetus's heart rate. This approach is thought to be simple and economical. Hence, in order to minimize fetal mortality and to detect fetal status early, it must be done by medical professionals. CTG results will track the mother's UC as well as the fetus's heart rate, acceleration events, series of decelerations, and other intricate measurements. The normal, suspicious, and pathological stages of the fetus can be classified

 DOI: 10.1201/9781003510932-6

using a variety of Machine Learning (ML) algorithms. The findings indicate that the ML approach will serve as a foundation for the automated system that analyzes the health of fetuses in the early stages.

6.2 LITERATURE SURVEY

Fetal health classification is a critical area in obstetrics, enabling early identification and management of potential health problems in unborn babies. ML has emerged as a promising tool for this task, offering the potential for automated and objective analysis of fetal health data. However, several challenges remain before widespread adoption in clinical practice. Several studies have explored different ML algorithms for fetal health classification using various data sources: A study analyzes the CTG data and compares three different models, i.e. extreme gradient boost, light gradient boost, and Support Vector Machines (SVMs); through their findings they proposed a novel algorithm based on randomized input sampling for explanation (RISE) called feature alteration for an explanation of black box models (FAB) [1].

They claimed that these methods can provide insight into the predictions of the black box model and help doctors and patients understand which features are most influential in the diagnosis of fetal health. Another research proposed a novel approach that enhances the accuracy, reliability, and comprehensiveness of fetal health assessment. The researchers present a LightGBM classifier [2] trained on a comprehensive dataset which achieved 98.31% accuracy considering various features, such as Fetal Heart Rate (FHR), UC, and maternal blood pressure. Their model offers a more holistic and reliable evaluation compared to traditional methods. Ultimately, Sujith K Mandala's work demonstrates the potential of ML in enhancing fetal health classification. Another study presents decision tree-based classification of fetal health using cardiotocograms (CTGs). The authors use the CART algorithm with the Gini index to analyze a dataset of 2126 CTG recordings and classify them into three classes: normal, suspect, or pathological. It reports a high accuracy of 93.65% for the decision tree model and suggests that it can be used as a medical decision support system for fetal health assessment. Weight is also an important feature of fetal health. Moreira et al. [3] used decision trees, SVMs, k-nearest neighbors, and ensemble learning methods to predict the fetal birth weight in high-risk pregnancies, especially those complicated by hypertensive disorders. The study showed ensemble learning methods, especially the bagged trees algorithm, achieved the best results. It further concluded that the ensemble learning methods are capable of efficiently predicting the expected weight of the fetus at birth. A similar study from Istanbul, Turkey proposes an e-health system that uses ML techniques to predict fetal health status based on maternal clinical history and evaluated nine binary classification algorithms [4] for their performance in predicting fetal anomalies. The best performing algorithm was decision forest, which achieved 89.5% accuracy. The study showed the impact of certain clinical data parameters of pregnancy on the fetal health status, statistically correlated the parameters with the existence of fetal anomalies, and showed guidelines for future research. Further investigating the use case of ML in fetal health classification, a study explored random forest, naïve Bayes, and SVM for the early prediction of fetal abnormalities based on

CTG data and compared the performance of the three classifiers using accuracy, sensitivity, specificity, and root mean square error (RMSE) metrics. It reported that random forest outperforms the other two classifiers with 99.93% accuracy and 0.1506 RMSE. Another recent study [5] evaluated ML models for predicting intrauterine growth restriction (IUGR) using a cross-sectional dataset from a tertiary hospital in Iran. They employed statistical learning algorithms such as decision tree classification, random forest classification, deep learning, and gradient boost algorithms. The study finds that deep learning has the best performance among the four models with an AUROC of 0.91, accuracy of 0.88, precision of 0.72, and sensitivity of 0.52. It further concluded that ML can accurately predict IUGR and emphasizes the importance of interpretability in model explanations. Deep neural networks also showed significant results to classify untapped pathological and suspicious CTG recordings with the desired time complexity as proposed by Muhammad et al. a hybrid deep learning model combining AlexNet and SVMs [6] on CTG data, achieving 99.72% accuracy, 96.67% sensitivity, and 99.6% specificity. Another study proposed a method to detect abnormalities based on deep learning techniques applied to ultrasound images [7]. It used three steps: finding the region of interest (ROI) of the fetal biometric and organ region in the ultrasound image using deep convolutional neural network (DCNN) models, evaluating the image quality by assessing the goodness of depiction for the key structures of fetal biometrics using AlexNet, GoogleNet, and CNN, and classifying the ultrasound images into normal or abnormal using the image quality scores. The method is tested on a dataset of 400 ultrasound images and achieves an accuracy of 90.43%, 88.70%, and 81.25% using AlexNet, GoogleNet, and CNN, respectively. A similar study utilized convolutional neural networks (CNN) and SVM [8], for estimating fetal weight and disease using ultrasound images, focusing on enhancing accuracy and aiding clinicians in identifying risks before delivery. It compares the results of multiclass SVM and CNN and finds that multiclass SVM outperforms CNN in terms of accuracy, sensitivity, specificity, and precision. The study concluded that the proposed model is effective and accurate in estimating fetal weight and disease using ultrasound images. Recent research has identified several challenges in fetal health classification using ML models applied to CTG data. These challenges impede the accurate interpretation of fetal health indicators and the development of robust classification models. Das et al. [9] and Salini et al. [10] outline some of the prevailing challenges: *Complex Fetal Heart Patterns*: CTG data presents intricate and dynamic patterns of fetal heart activity, making accurate interpretation challenging for both visual and automated methods [11]. *Limited Interpretation Accuracy*: Despite advancements in CTG analysis automation, the accuracy of interpretation remains low, particularly in suspected cases, posing risks for misdiagnosis or delayed intervention. *Distinct Fetal Heart Rate Dynamics*: The different stages of labor produce significantly different FHR dynamics, necessitating separate consideration for accurate classification [12]. *Data Complexity*: CTG data is inherently complex, requiring sophisticated approaches for feature extraction and classification to capture meaningful information [13]. *Limited Labeled Samples*: The availability of labeled samples for training and validation is scarce, hindering the development of accurate and robust classification models [14]. *Data Availability and Quality*: Freely available CTG datasets are often small and may not fully represent the diversity and complexity of real-world scenarios. Preprocessing and feature engineering are necessary to enhance data quality and informativeness [15]. *Model Selection and Evaluation*: The chapter compares various ML models and evaluates their performance using multiple metrics. Considerations include model complexity, interpretability, and generalizability, as well as trade-offs between different algorithms [16]. *Clinical Integration and Adoption*: ML models are intended to assist rather than replace clinical judgment. Challenges include validation, integration into clinical workflows, regulatory compliance, user-friendliness, and ethical considerations. As technology evolves and datasets expand, future research endeavors should focus on addressing the identified challenges, such as improving interpretability, enhancing data quality, and refining model evaluation techniques. Additionally, exploring novel data sources and integrating multimodal data could provide deeper insights into fetal health assessment. Ultimately, the successful integration of ML into fetal health classification has the potential to revolutionize prenatal care by enabling earlier detection of fetal anomalies, personalized risk assessment, and optimized clinical decision-making.

6.3 PROPOSED METHODOLOGY

A woman is happiest during her pregnancy. Given that she is carrying a child, a mother needs to take extra care of her health during pregnancy. There are several recommended laboratory tests per trimester to track fetal growth and development. The CTG, which is frequently used in clinical evaluation to assess the fetus's health inside the uterus, is one of the tests, employing the two CTG signals of UC and FHR for prenatal monitoring. Preterm birth can be avoided, and the risk of perinatal death can be decreased using CTG results. Although medical experts are trying to develop an automated CTG interpretation, the results have not been able to identify any suspicious fetal abnormalities. Data on fetal health undergoes a variety of algorithmic preparation steps before modeling. Based on the input parameters, the resulting model is used in the interface to verify fetal growth. With the aid of this interface which is in Figure 6.1, expectant mothers will be able to monitor their fetal growth on a daily basis. Women can quickly and easily get in touch with a doctor in an emergency.

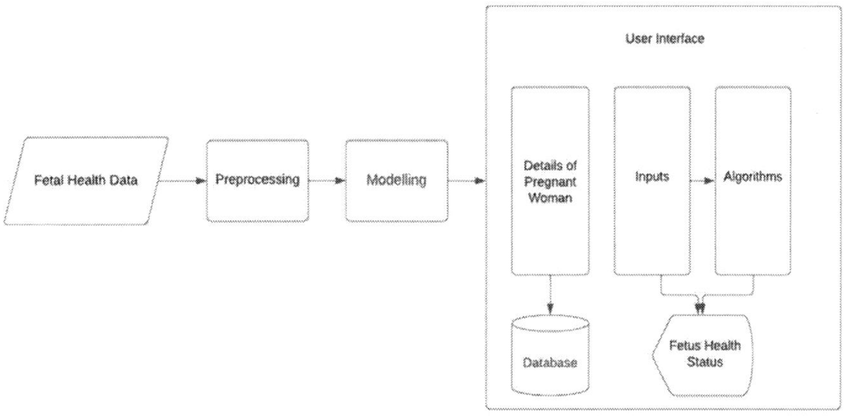

FIGURE 6.1 Interface to check fetal growth.

TABLE 6.1
Features in the Dataset

baseline_value	acceleration	fetal_movement	uterine_contractions	light_decelerations
severe_ decelerations	prolonged_ decelerations	abnormal_ short_term_ variability	mean_value_of_ short_term_ variability	percentage_of_ time_with_ abnormal_long_ term_variability
histogram_ number_of_ peaks	histogram_ width	histogram_min	histogram_max	mean_value_of_ long_term_ variability
histogram_ variance	histogram_ mode	histogram_ mean	histogram_median	histogram_ number_of_ zeroes
histogram_ tendency	fetal_health			

6.3.1 About Dataset

This fetal health classification was collected from the University of California Irvine ML Repository consisting of 2126 data of pregnant ladies in their third trimester. It uses CTG data. This dataset consists of FHR and UC which helps to determine the fetal health (normal, suspect, or pathological). The different features are shown in Table 6.1.

The heat map for the various features has been presented in Figure 6.2.

Different plots have been drawn corresponding to various features, as shown in Figure 6.3.

6.4 MACHINE LEARNING MODELS

6.4.1 KNN

KNN stands out as one of the classification methods in the field of ML. It falls under the category of supervised learning. It is extensively used in tasks such as recognizing patterns, mining data, and detecting outliers. Its practicality in real-world situations is notable due to its parametric nature. It doesn't rely on specific assumptions about data distribution like some other algorithms such as GMM do with assuming a Gaussian distribution. There are several ways to measure the distance between the nodes like Euclidean distance (Eq. 6.1) and Manhattan distance metric, as shown in Eq. (6.2).

$$distance(\alpha,\beta)=\sum_{d=1}^{n}(\beta_d-\alpha_d)^2, \tag{6.1}$$

$$distance(\alpha,\beta)=\sum_{d=1}^{n}\|\beta_d-\alpha_d\|. \tag{6.2}$$

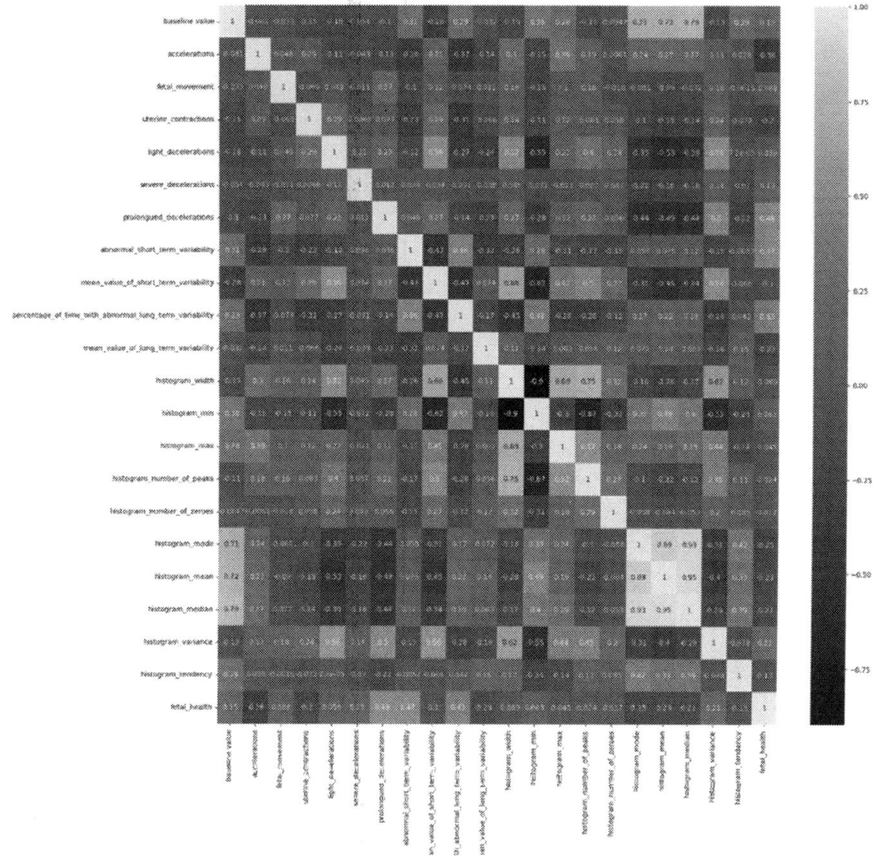

FIGURE 6.2 Heat map for different features.

6.4.2 Random Forest

The random forest algorithm stands out as a tree-based learning method, within the realm of ML. It operates by generating decision trees in the training phase with each tree being built using a subset of the dataset to evaluate a random subset of features within each partition. This element of randomness adds diversity among trees reducing the risk of overfitting and enhancing accuracy. During prediction, the algorithm consolidates the outcomes from all trees through voting (for classification tasks) and averaging (for regression tasks). This collaborative decision-making approach, driven by trees and their unique perspectives, yields precise results [17].

6.4.3 SVM (Support Vector Machine)

The SVM is a machine learning technique which is used for classification and regression tasks. While it can handle regression problems, SVM is most effective for classification purposes. Its primary goal is to determine the hyperplane in an N space to separate data points into distinct classes within the feature space. The hyperplane aims to maximize

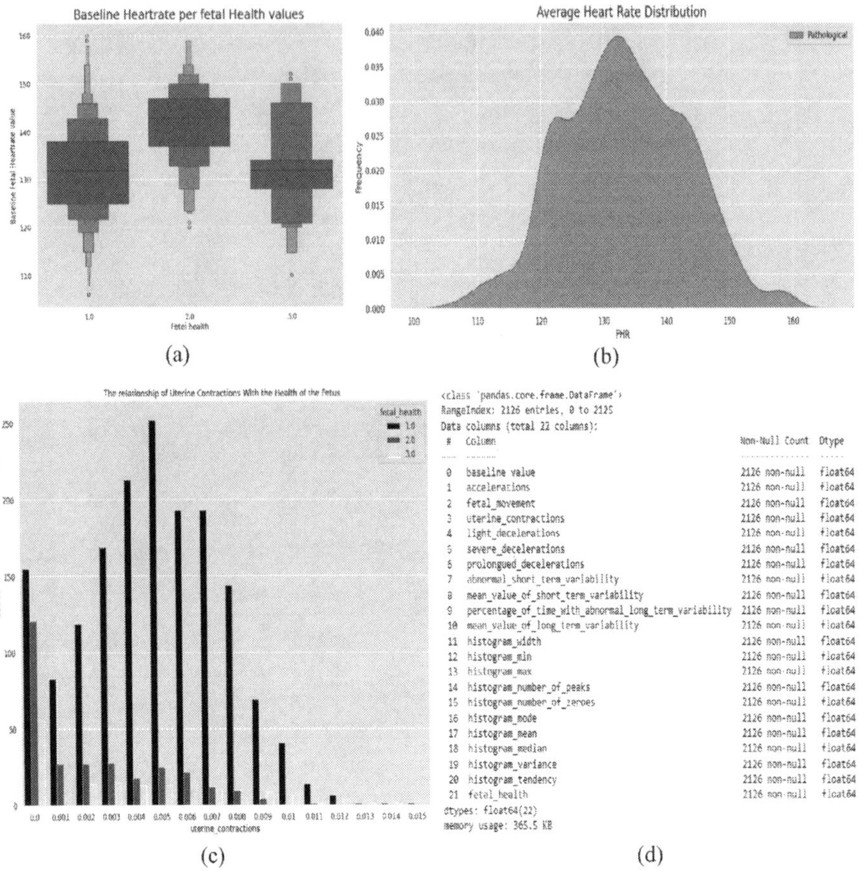

FIGURE 6.3 (a) Baseline heart rate per fetal health values; (b) average heart rate distribution; (c) relationship between uterine contraction with the health of the fetus; (d) data types of the various features.

the margin between the points of classes [18]. The dimension of the hyperplane is determined by the number of features: with two features, it forms a line; with three features, a 2D plane; and with more than three features, visualization becomes increasingly difficult.

6.4.4 Decision Tree

A decision tree resembles a flowchart with branches representing rules, internal nodes denoting features, and leaf nodes showing the algorithm's outcome. This versatile supervised ML method is applied to solve classification and regression challenges making it an effective algorithm. It can be used for both classification and regression tasks. The original dataset is divided into subsets using attribute selection measures to create a tree. These measures are criteria used in decision tree algorithms to assess the importance of attributes, in splitting the data. The aim is to find the attribute that leads to the subsets of data after splitting and maximizing information gain. This process continues recursively on each subset until all nodes have identical target variable values or further splitting does not improve predictions. Building a decision tree classifier does not necessitate domain knowledge or parameter adjustments, making it suitable for discovering insights. Decision trees are effective at handling data with dimensions [19].

6.4.5 Logistic Regression

Logistic regression is commonly employed in scenarios involving classification. It utilizes a sigmoid function that considers variables as input and generates a probability ranging from 0 to 1. Logistic function with sigmoid function is shown in Eq. (6.3) [20].

$$\alpha(p) = \frac{1}{1 - exp^{-p}}. \tag{6.3}$$

6.5 RESULTS AND DISCUSSIONS

6.5.1 Classification Models

Different classification models like KNN, SVM (linear, polynomial, RBF), logistic regression, and decision tree have been applied to the dataset. As desired, accuracy has not been achieved. So, the feature selection process was imposed on the dataset, and then random forest was applied to ten relevant features that were highly correlated to fetal health, and an accuracy of 93.06% was achieved.

The selected features were baseline_value, prolonged_decelerations, histogram_mode, mean_value_of_long_term_variability, histogram_median, histogram_mean, accelerations, mean_value_of_short_term_variability, percentage of time with abnormal long-term variability, abnormal short-term variability.

The performance of various ML models used to classify fetal health status based on CTG data has been shown based on several metrics like accuracy, precision, recall, and F1-score, which is shown in Table 6.2. Out of all, random forest performs the best and provides the highest accuracy of 93.06%.

TABLE 6.2
Performance Metrics

S. No.	Model	Accuracy	Precision Score	Recall Score	F1 Score	Sensitivity
1	KNN	88.4	88.7	86.95	87.72	86.95
2	Logistic regression	47.97	53.90	54.61	45.91	54.61
3	Decision tree	89.01	88.70	88.95	88.80	88.95
4	**Random forest**	**93.06**	**92.53**	**94.09**	**93.18**	**94.09**
5	Linear SVM	80.92	81.02	79.81	80.26	79.81
6	Polynomial SVM	79.76	79.22	78.74	78.90	78.74
7	RBF SVM	47.39	73.80	35.95	26.11	35.95

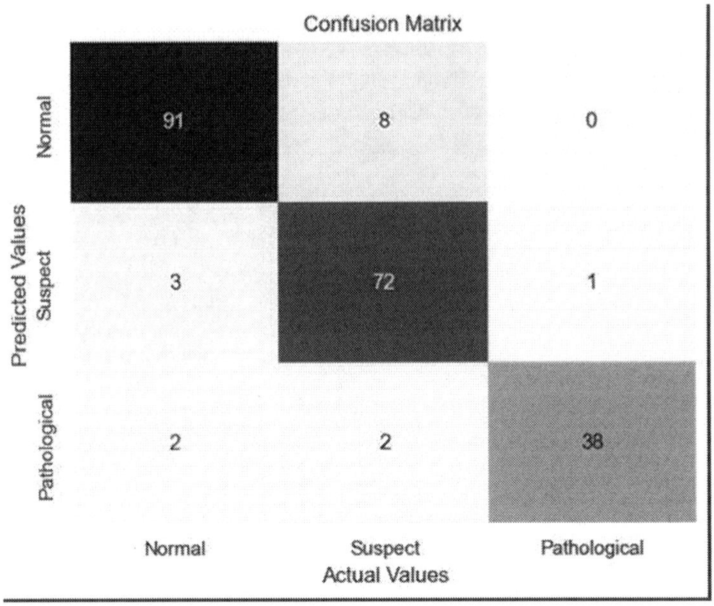

FIGURE 6.4 Confusion matrix for random forest.

The confusion matrices for random forest have been shown in Figure 6.4.

6.5.2 Interface for Tracking Pregnant Women's Fetal Health Conditions

The best prediction model found by analyzing the dataset is fed into the backend of the interface to predict fetal health. Figure 6.5 shows the interface for tracking

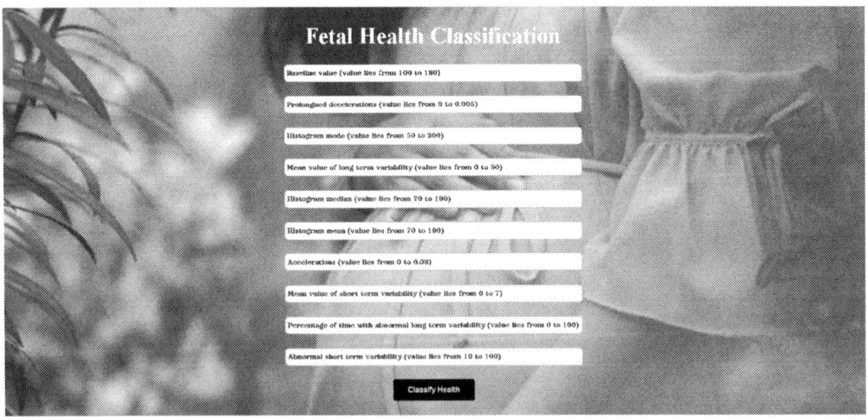

FIGURE 6.5 Interface for tracking the fetus's health.

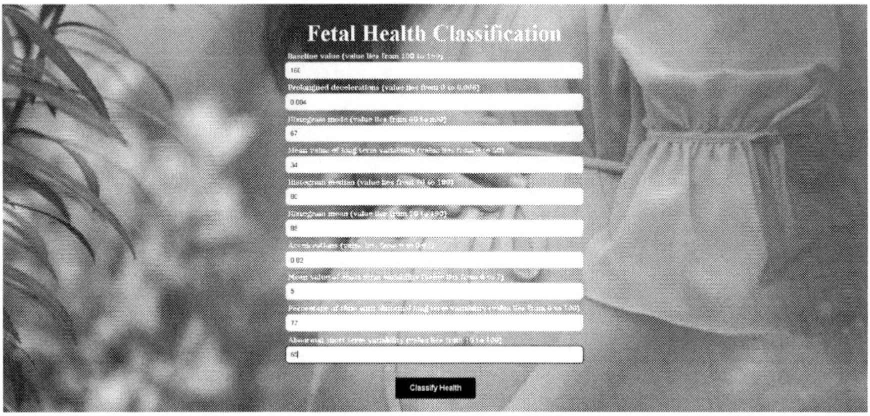

FIGURE 6.6 After inserting the values.

the health of the fetus of a pregnant woman, after feeding the input values into the interface as shown in Figure 6.6.

After submitting the inputs, the fetus's health can lie in any of the three classes (normal, suspect, and pathological). Figures 6.7–6.9 show each of the result categories. The result page also includes the recommendation for a particular class.

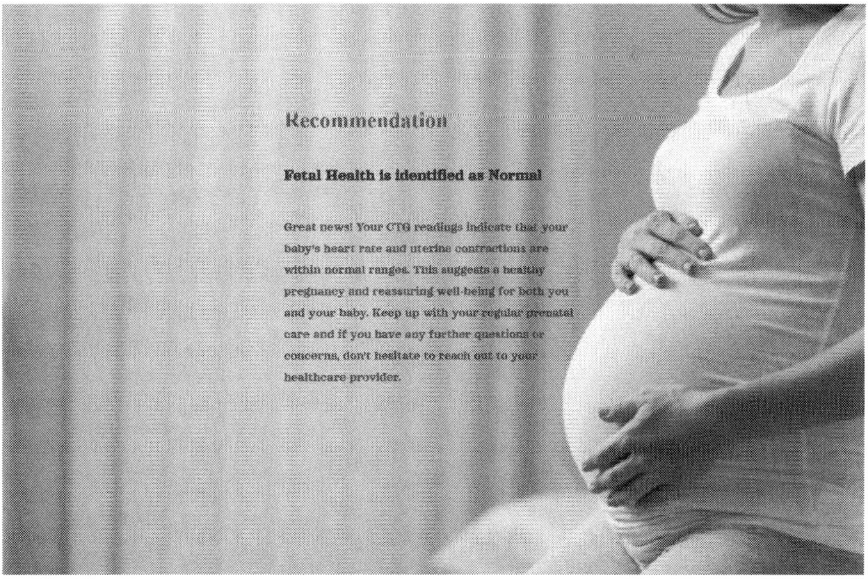

FIGURE 6.7 Result page for normal.

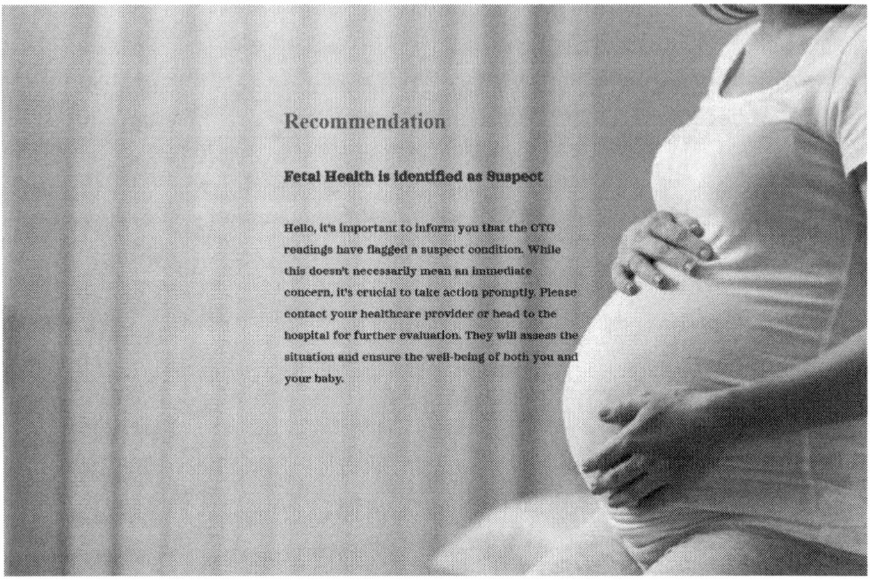

FIGURE 6.8 Result page for suspect.

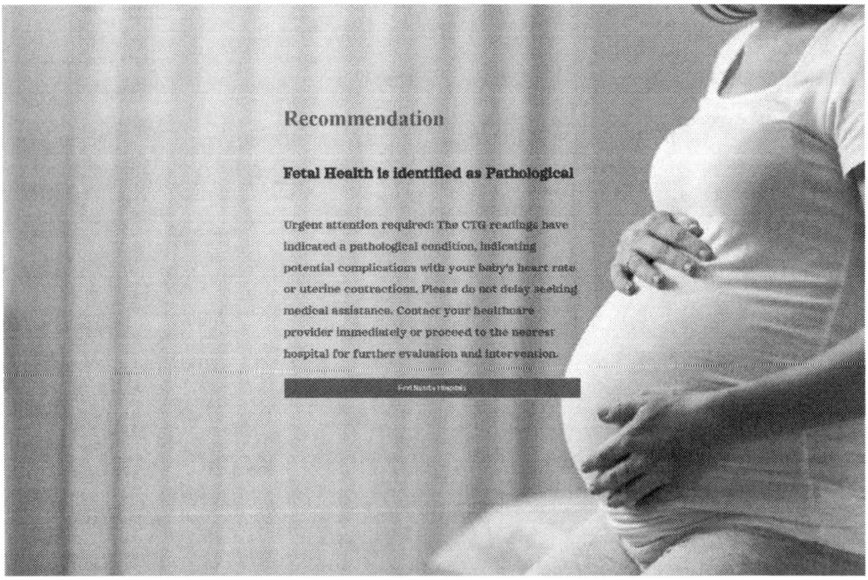

FIGURE 6.9 Result page for pathological.

6.6 CONCLUSION AND FUTURE WORK

The interface for monitoring fetal health conditions based on CTG information categorizes outputs into normal, suspect, and pathological, aiding in early detection and interventions. Our model accurately predicts normal, suspect, and pathological cases, showcasing its potential to improve maternal and fetal healthcare. Embracing technological advancements like this interface can significantly improve outcomes for pregnant women and their unborn children.

REFERENCES

1. Yin, Y., & Bingi, Y. (2023). Using machine learning to classify human fetal health and analyze feature importance. *BioMedInformatics*, *3*(2), 280–298.
2. Mandala, S. K. (2023). Unveiling the unborn: Advancing fetal health classification through machine learning. *arXiv preprint arXiv:2310.00505*.
3. Moreira, M. W., Rodrigues, J. J., Furtado, V., Mavromoustakis, C. X., Kumar, N., & Woungang, I. (2019, May). Fetal birth weight estimation in high-risk pregnancies through machine learning techniques. In *ICC 2019-2019 IEEE International Conference on Communications (ICC)* (pp. 1–6). IEEE.
4. Akbulut, A., Ertugrul, E., & Topcu, V. (2018). Fetal health status prediction based on maternal clinical history using machine learning techniques. *Computer Methods and Programs in Biomedicine*, *163*, 87–100.
5. Taeidi, E., Ranjbar, A., Montazeri, F., Mehrnoush, V., & Darsareh, F. (2023). Machine learning-based approach to predict intrauterine growth restriction. *Cureus*, *15*(7).
6. Muhammad Hussain, N., Rehman, A. U., Othman, M. T. B., Zafar, J., Zafar, H., & Hamam, H. (2022). Accessing artificial intelligence for fetus health status using hybrid deep learning algorithm (AlexNet-SVM) on cardiotocographic data. *Sensors*, *22*(14), 5103.
7. Selvathi, D., & Chandralekha, R. (2022). Fetal biometric based abnormality detection during prenatal development using deep learning techniques. *Multidimensional Systems and Signal Processing*, *33*(1), 1–15.
8. Bijapur, S. (2023). An approach for fetal weight estimation using machine learning for women safety. *Journal of Scientific Research and Technology*, *1*(6), 136–144.
9. Das, S., Mukherjee, H., Roy, K., & Saha, C. K. (2023). Fetal health classification from cardiotocograph for both stages of labor—A soft-computing-based approach. *Diagnostics*, *13*(5), 858.
10. Salini, Y., Mohanty, S. N., Ramesh, J. V. N., Yang, M., & Chalapathi, M. M. V. (2024). Cardiotocography data analysis for fetal health classification using machine learning models. *IEEE Access*, *12*, 26005–26022.
11. Han, Q., Qian, X., Xu, H., Wu, K., Meng, L., Qiu, Z., … & Gao, X. (2024). DM-CNN: Dynamic multi-scale convolutional neural network with uncertainty quantification for medical image classification. *Computers in Biology and Medicine*, *168*, 107758.
12. Krishna, T. B., & Kokil, P. (2024). Standard fetal ultrasound plane classification based on stacked ensemble of deep learning models. *Expert Systems with Applications*, *238*, 122153.
13. Berezsky, O., Liashchynskyi, P., Pitsun, O., & Izonin, I. (2024). Synthesis of convolutional neural network architectures for biomedical image classification. *Biomedical Signal Processing and Control*, *95*, 106325.
14. Al-Razgan, M., Ali, Y. A., & Awwad, E. M. (2024). Enhancing fetal medical image analysis through attention-guided convolution: A comparative study with established models. *Journal of Disability Research*, *3*(2), 20240005.

15. Liu, L., Tang, D., Li, X., & Ouyang, Y. (2024). Automatic fetal ultrasound image segmentation of first trimester for measuring biometric parameters based on deep learning. *Multimedia Tools and Applications*, *83*(9), 27283–27304.
16. Archana, R., & Jeevaraj, P. E. (2024). Deep learning models for digital image processing: A review. *Artificial Intelligence Review*, *57*(1), 11.
17. Mavaluru, D., Ravula, S. R., Auguskani, J. P. L., Dharmarajlu, S. M., Chellathurai, A., Ramakrishnan, J., … & Ravishankar, N. (2024). Advancing fetal ultrasound diagnostics: Innovative methodologies for improved accuracy in detecting down syndrome. *Medical Engineering & Physics*, 104132.
18. Kumar, R., Kumbharkar, P., Vanam, S., & Sharma, S. (2024). Medical images classification using deep learning: A survey. *Multimedia Tools and Applications*, *83*(7), 19683–19728.
19. Francis, F., Luz, S., Wu, H., Stock, S. J., & Townsend, R. (2024). Machine learning on cardiotocography data to classify fetal outcomes: A scoping review. *Computers in Biology and Medicine*, volume 172 108220.
20. Breesha, S. R., & Vinsley, S. S. (2024). Automated extraction of fetal ECG signal features using twinned filter and integrated methodologies. *Circuits, Systems, and Signal Processing*, *43*(2), 661–683.

7 Blockchain for Medical Data Management

Ensuring Integrity and Accessibility

Ambika Aggarwal and Ashutosh Bhatt

7.1 INTRODUCTION

In the modern digital world, data has become the keystone of many industries, and healthcare is no exception. Medical data, which includes patient records, clinical trial results, imaging data, genomic sequences, and other health-related information, is critical to the functioning of healthcare systems. This data enables healthcare providers to diagnose, treat, and monitor patients effectively, and it supports the ongoing development of medical research and public health initiatives [1]. However, the growing volume and complexity of medical data have brought up significant challenges in terms of management, security, and accessibility. Medical data management refers to the processes and systems used for collecting, storing, organizing, retrieving, and analyzing health information. The transition from paper-based records to digital systems has brought immense benefits, such as improving the efficiency of healthcare delivery, enabling remote consultations, and facilitating big data analytics in medical research. Nevertheless, this digital shift has also exposed vulnerabilities, particularly in terms of data security, privacy, and interoperability between different healthcare systems. Centralized databases, which are commonly used for storing medical records, have become prime targets for cyberattacks, and data breaches have become a growing concern [2]. Figure 7.1 presents the role of blockchain in healthcare.

The healthcare sector is particularly vulnerable to data breaches due to the sensitive nature of the information it handles. Personal health information (PHI) is not only valuable to hackers but is also difficult to replace or recover once it is compromised [3]. The impact of a data breach on healthcare extends beyond financial loss; it can also decline patient trust, lead to identity theft, and in some cases, even result in medical errors or compromised care. In light of these risks, there is an urgent need for more secure and resilient systems for managing medical data.

Enter blockchain technology—a decentralized, distributed ledger system originally developed to support digital currencies like Bitcoin. Over the past decade, blockchain has evolved beyond its financial roots and has been

DOI: 10.1201/9781003510932-7

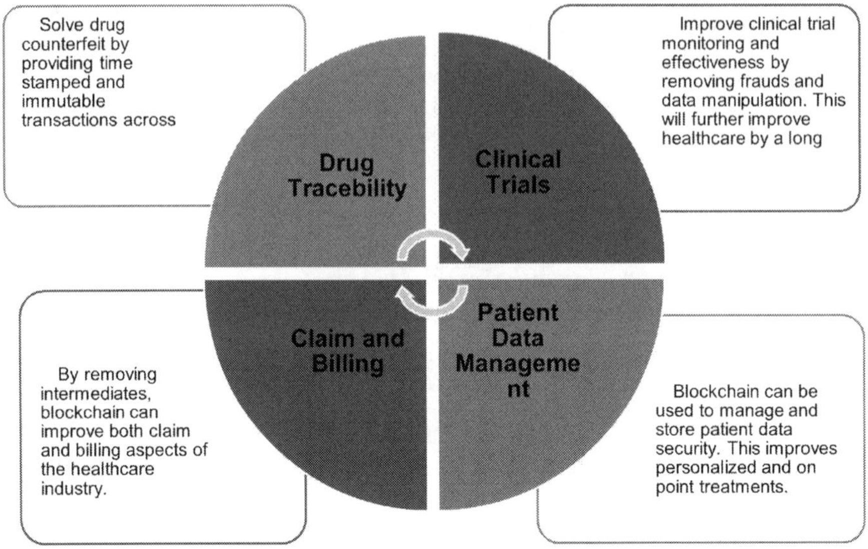

FIGURE 7.1 Blockchain in healthcare.

recognized as a potential solution for the data management challenges faced by various industries, including healthcare. By decentralizing the storage of data and securing it through cryptographic algorithms, blockchain offers a new paradigm for managing medical information that promises to enhance security, integrity, and accessibility. Blockchain's unique architecture provides several key advantages over traditional centralized systems. At its core, blockchain operates as a distributed ledger, where each transaction (or "block") is recorded in a chain that is replicated across multiple nodes in a network. This decentralized structure makes blockchain inherently resistant to tampering and unauthorized access. Because there is no central point of failure, hackers would need to compromise a majority of the nodes in the network simultaneously to alter the data, a feat that is practically impossible in a well-maintained blockchain [4].

Moreover, blockchain uses cryptographic techniques to ensure that data remains secure and private. Each block in the chain is linked to the previous one using a cryptographic hash, and transactions are validated through consensus mechanisms, such as Proof of Work (PoW) or Proof of Stake (PoS). This ensures that once data is recorded in the blockchain, it cannot be altered without detection. For medical data, this immutability is crucial—it means that patient records, clinical trial data, and other health information can be trusted as accurate and untampered with [5].

Besides security, blockchain also addresses issues of data accessibility and patient control over data. Traditional centralized databases are often siloed, meaning that patient data is scattered across multiple healthcare providers, making it difficult to obtain a comprehensive view of a patient's medical history [6]. This fragmentation can lead to inefficiencies, such as redundant tests or delayed diagnoses, and can increase the risk of medical errors. Blockchain, on the other hand, allows for the creation of a unified, decentralized database that can be accessed by authorized parties in real time. This has the potential to improve the quality of care by ensuring that healthcare providers have access to the most up-to-date and complete information.

Importantly, blockchain also empowers patients by giving them greater control over their health data. In traditional systems, patients often had little visibility or control over who accessed their information. Blockchain can change this by enabling patients to decide who can view their data and for how long. With the help of cryptographic keys, patients can grant and revoke access to their information as needed, ensuring that their privacy is respected. The promise of blockchain in healthcare extends beyond just security and accessibility. It also has the potential to facilitate interoperability between different healthcare systems, which has long been a challenge in the industry. Today, healthcare providers use a variety of electronic health record (EHR) systems, each with its own proprietary standards for storing and exchanging data. This lack of standardization makes it difficult for providers to share patient information across different systems, leading to inefficiencies and delays in care. Blockchain, with its decentralized nature and standardized protocols, can serve as a bridge between these disparate systems, enabling seamless data exchange and enhancing the continuity of care [7].

However, the adoption of blockchain in healthcare is not without challenges. The technology is still relatively new, and there are technical, regulatory, and operational hurdles to overcome before it can be widely implemented. Blockchain networks, especially public ones, face scalability issues—they can only process a limited number of transactions per second, which may not be sufficient for the high volume of data generated by the healthcare industry. Additionally, integrating blockchain with existing healthcare IT infrastructure can be complex and costly. There are also legal and ethical considerations, particularly regarding data privacy and compliance with regulations like the Health Insurance Portability and Accountability Act (HIPAA) in the United States and the General Data Protection Regulation (GDPR) in Europe [8].

Despite these challenges, the potential benefits of blockchain for medical data management are significant. As technology continues to mature, it is expected to play an increasingly important role in the future of healthcare. Blockchain has the power to revolutionize the way medical data is stored, shared, and protected, leading to a more secure, efficient, and patient-centered healthcare system [9].

In this chapter, we will explore the various ways in which blockchain can be applied to medical data management. We will examine the current state of medical data management systems and the challenges they face, discuss the advantages of blockchain technology in addressing these challenges, and present real-world case studies of blockchain implementations in healthcare. Finally, we will consider the future of blockchain in healthcare and the steps needed to overcome the obstacles to its adoption.

- *The State of Medical Data Management Today*

  Medical data management is one of the most critical aspects of healthcare delivery in the modern world. The effective handling of patient information, diagnostic records, treatment histories, and other health-related data is essential for the proper functioning of healthcare systems. However, the current state of medical data management faces numerous challenges that threaten both the quality of care and the security of patient information. Understanding the landscape of existing systems and their shortcomings is crucial to appreciating the potential of blockchain as a transformative solution [10].
- *The Evolution of Medical Data Management*

  Historically, medical data management relied on paper-based systems, where patient records were stored in physical files within healthcare facilities. These systems were prone to a range of issues, including loss of records, difficulty in retrieving information, and errors in data entry. Moreover, sharing patient data between different providers was a cumbersome and time-consuming process that often required physical transfers or lengthy communications. The digitization of healthcare records, driven by the adoption of EHRs systems, marked a significant improvement. EHR systems allow for the digital storage of patient information, making it easier for healthcare providers to access and share data [10]. With EHRs, physicians could quickly pull up a patient's medical history, lab results, and treatment plans, leading to more informed decision-making and improved patient outcomes. Furthermore, digital records enabled the analysis of large datasets to identify trends, optimize treatment protocols, and contribute to medical research. Despite these advancements, the digitization of medical data introduced a new set of challenges. The centralized nature of many EHR systems made them vulnerable to cyberattacks, and interoperability issues between different systems hindered the seamless sharing of information across the healthcare ecosystem [10]. Additionally, concerns about data privacy and security have become increasingly prominent as healthcare data breaches have become more frequent and damaging.

7.2 CURRENT CHALLENGES IN MEDICAL DATA MANAGEMENT

Medical data management faces several significant challenges that impact the healthcare industry's ability to securely, efficiently, and effectively handle patient data. Figure 7.2 presents some of the key challenges in this domain [10].

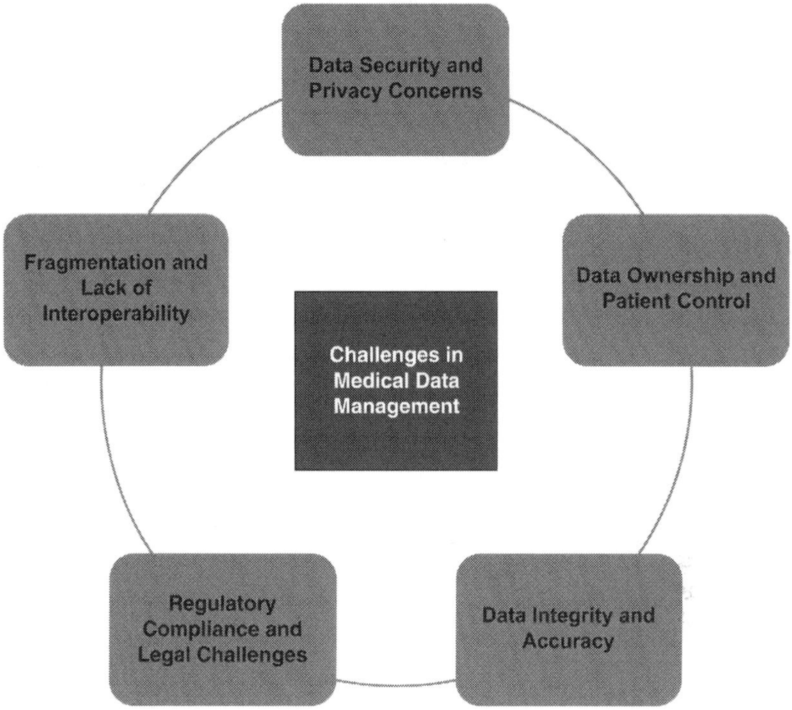
Data Security and Privacy Concerns
Data Ownership and Patient Control
Data Integrity and Accuracy
Regulatory Compliance and Legal Challenges
Fragmentation and Lack of Interoperability
Challenges in Medical Data Management

FIGURE 7.2 Challenges in medical data management.

7.3 FRAGMENTATION AND LACK OF INTEROPERABILITY

One of the most important issues in medical data management today is the fragmentation of data across different healthcare systems. While the adoption of EHRs has improved data storage and accessibility within individual healthcare providers, it has also led to the creation of data silos. These silos exist because different healthcare providers often use incompatible systems that cannot communicate with each other effectively.

For example, a patient who visits multiple healthcare providers—such as a general practitioner, a specialist, and a hospital—might have their medical data stored in separate EHR systems [11]. These systems may use different formats and protocols, making it difficult or impossible for one provider to access the data from another. As a result, providers often do not have a complete view of a patient's medical history, leading to inefficiencies, delays in care, and the potential for medical errors. The lack of interoperability between healthcare systems also hinders the ability to aggregate and analyze data for research purposes. Large-scale studies that require data from multiple sources are often hampered by the challenges of merging datasets from different systems. This fragmentation not only impacts patient care but also limits the potential for advancements in medical research and public health initiatives.

7.4 DATA SECURITY AND PRIVACY CONCERNS

Healthcare data is among the most sensitive types of information, containing personal details such as medical histories, diagnoses, treatment plans, and genetic information. Protecting this data from unauthorized access and breaches is a top priority for healthcare organizations. However, the healthcare industry has become a prime target for cybercriminals due to the value of medical data on the black market [12]. According to a study by IBM Security, the average cost of a data breach in the healthcare sector was $10.93 million in 2023, the highest across all industries. Centralized EHR systems are particularly vulnerable to cyberattacks. These systems often house vast amounts of sensitive data in a single location, making them attractive targets for hackers. A successful breach can expose the personal information of thousands or even millions of patients, leading to identity theft, financial fraud, and other forms of exploitation. In some cases, cyberattacks have also disrupted healthcare operations, forcing hospitals to shut down systems and delay critical care [13].

In addition to external threats, healthcare organizations must also deal with internal risks. Data breaches can also occur due to human error, such as employees accidentally sharing sensitive information or falling victim to phishing attacks. Insider threats, where employees intentionally misuse their access to data for personal gain, also pose a significant risk.

To address these challenges, healthcare organizations have implemented various security measures, including encryption, firewalls, and multi-factor authentication. However, these measures are not foolproof, and breaches continue to occur. Moreover, ensuring compliance with data privacy regulations, such as the HIPAA in the United States and the GDPR in Europe, adds another layer of complexity to data management efforts [14].

7.5 DATA OWNERSHIP AND PATIENT CONTROL

One of the ongoing debates in medical data management revolves around the issue of data ownership. In many healthcare systems, patients have little control over their health data once it is collected by a healthcare provider. Although patients may have the right to access their records, the actual data is often stored and managed by the provider or a third-party vendor. This lack of control can lead to situations where patients are unaware of how their data is being used or who has access to it. The lack of transparency in data handling can erode patient trust in healthcare providers and the broader healthcare system. For example, patients may be concerned about their data being shared with insurance companies, employers, or pharmaceutical companies without their explicit consent. In some cases, patients may be hesitant to share important health information with their providers due to fears about how the data might be used or disclosed.

Furthermore, the process of accessing one's medical data can be cumbersome and time-consuming. Patients often have to go through lengthy procedures to obtain copies of their records, and in some cases, they may be charged fees for access. This lack of easy access to data can be particularly problematic for patients who need to share their health information with new providers or who require access to their records for personal use. The concept of patient-centered care, which emphasizes the importance of involving patients in their healthcare decisions, is gaining traction. However, achieving true patient-centered care requires giving patients greater control over their data. This includes the ability to decide who can access their information and for what purposes, as well as the ability to revoke access when needed. Empowering patients with control over their data can improve trust, enhance the quality of care, and facilitate more effective communication between patients and providers.

7.6 DATA INTEGRITY AND ACCURACY

Ensuring the integrity and accuracy of medical data is very important for providing high-quality care. Inaccurate or incomplete data can lead to misdiagnoses, inappropriate treatments, and medical errors that can have serious consequences for patients. However, maintaining data integrity is challenging, especially in systems where data is entered manually by healthcare providers. Human error is a significant factor in data inaccuracies. For example, a provider might inadvertently enter the wrong dosage for a medication or record an incorrect diagnosis. These errors can propagate throughout the healthcare system, affecting treatment decisions and patient outcomes. In some cases, data can be lost or corrupted during transfers between systems, leading to gaps in a patient's medical history. Data integrity is also affected by the sheer volume of information that healthcare providers must manage. As new technologies, such as wearable devices and remote monitoring tools, generate vast amounts of real-time health data, the challenge of ensuring that all of this information is accurately recorded and integrated into a patient's record becomes even more complex. To mitigate these risks, healthcare organizations have implemented various quality control measures, such as data validation protocols and regular audits of medical records. However, these processes can be time-consuming and resource-intensive, and they are not always sufficient to prevent errors.

7.7 REGULATORY COMPLIANCE AND LEGAL CHALLENGES

Healthcare organizations are subject to a range of regulatory requirements related to data privacy, security, and management. In the United States, HIPAA sets the standards for protecting sensitive patient information, while in Europe, the GDPR imposes strict rules on how personal data, including health data, can be collected, stored, and used. Non-compliance with these regulations can result in significant fines, legal liabilities, and reputational damage. Navigating the complex web of regulatory requirements can be challenging for healthcare providers, especially as regulations evolve in response to new threats and technological developments. For example, the GDPR includes provisions that give individuals the right to be forgotten, meaning that they can request the deletion of their personal data from an organization's systems. Implementing such requests in a way that complies with the regulation while maintaining the integrity of medical records is a difficult balancing act for healthcare providers.

In addition to data privacy regulations, healthcare organizations must also comply with industry-specific standards related to the management of medical information.

These standards, such as the Health Level Seven (HL7) standards for electronic health data exchange, are designed to ensure that data is handled consistently and securely across different systems. However, keeping up with these standards and ensuring that systems are compliant can be a significant burden for healthcare organizations, particularly smaller providers with limited resources. The current state of medical data management is fraught with challenges that impact the security, accessibility, and integrity of patient information. Centralized systems, while a significant improvement over paper-based records, have shown vulnerabilities in terms of data fragmentation, security risks, and limited patient control. The healthcare industry is at a crossroads, where the limitations of traditional systems are becoming increasingly apparent, and the need for innovative solutions is more pressing than ever. Blockchain technology offers a promising alternative that addresses many of the shortcomings of existing medical data management systems. By decentralizing data storage, enhancing security through cryptography, and empowering patients with control over their data, blockchain has the potential to revolutionize the way medical information is managed and shared across the healthcare ecosystem. The next sections of this chapter will delve into how blockchain can overcome these challenges and transform the future of healthcare data management.

7.8 THE BLOCKCHAIN ADVANTAGE: DECENTRALIZATION, SECURITY, AND TRANSPARENCY

Blockchain technology has emerged as a ground-breaking innovation with the potential to transform various industries, and healthcare is no exception. Its decentralized, secure, and transparent architecture addresses some of the most pressing challenges in medical data management, including data fragmentation, security vulnerabilities, and lack of transparency [15]. By leveraging blockchain, healthcare systems can enhance the integrity, accessibility, and privacy of medical data, ultimately improving patient care and empowering individuals with control over their health information. This section delves deeper into the key advantages of blockchain technology—decentralization, security, and transparency—and explores how these features can reshape medical data management.

- *Decentralization*: At the heart of blockchain technology is its decentralized structure, which fundamentally changes how data is stored, managed, and accessed. Traditional medical data management systems rely on centralized databases, where data is stored in a single location or controlled by a single entity, such as a healthcare provider, hospital, or third-party service. While centralized systems have been the norm for decades, they present several challenges, including the risk of data breaches, single points of failure, and limited interoperability. Blockchain, by contrast, operates as a decentralized, distributed ledger system. In a blockchain network, data is not stored in a single location but is distributed across multiple nodes (computers) that participate in the network. Each node contains a copy of the entire blockchain, which is continuously updated as new transactions (or "blocks") are added to the chain. This decentralized approach offers several key advantages over traditional centralized systems.

- *Resilience and Redundancy*: In a decentralized blockchain network, data is replicated across all participating nodes. This means that even if one or several nodes fail or are compromised, the rest of the network remains operational, ensuring that data is not lost or inaccessible. This redundancy makes blockchain networks inherently more resilient to failures and attacks than centralized systems, where a single breach or technical failure can disrupt the entire system.
- *Elimination of Single Points of Failure*: Centralized systems are vulnerable to single points of failure, where a breach or failure at a central server can compromise the entire database. In contrast, blockchain's decentralized architecture distributes risk across the network [16]. To alter or tamper with data on a blockchain, an attacker would need to compromise the majority of the network's nodes simultaneously—a task that becomes exponentially more difficult as the network grows larger and more distributed.
- *Enhanced Interoperability*: Decentralization also facilitates interoperability between different healthcare systems. In traditional centralized systems, data is often siloed within individual organizations, making it difficult to share information across different providers and platforms. Blockchain's decentralized ledger can serve as a universal, shared platform where authorized participants can securely access and share data. This can help bridge the gap between disparate EHR systems and enable more seamless data exchange across the healthcare ecosystem.
- *Patient Empowerment and Control*: Decentralization also aligns with the growing movement toward patient-centered care. In traditional systems, patients have limited control over their medical data, which is often stored and managed by healthcare providers or third-party vendors. Blockchain empowers patients by allowing them to control access to their data. With the use of cryptographic keys, patients can grant or revoke access to specific pieces of their health information, ensuring that only authorized parties can view or use their data. This decentralization of data ownership gives patients more autonomy over their health information and enhances trust in the healthcare system [16].

7.9 SECURITY: SAFEGUARDING MEDICAL DATA WITH CRYPTOGRAPHY

One of the most critical advantages of blockchain technology is its robust security features, which are designed to protect data from unauthorized access, tampering, and breaches. Security is a paramount concern in healthcare, where sensitive medical information must be protected to ensure patient privacy and comply with regulatory requirements. Blockchain addresses many of the security vulnerabilities associated with traditional centralized systems through its use of cryptography and consensus mechanisms.

- *Immutability and Tamper Resistance*: Once data is recorded on a blockchain, it is virtually impossible to alter or delete without the consensus of the network. Each block in the blockchain contains a cryptographic hash of the previous block, creating a chain of blocks that are linked together. If an attacker attempts to alter the data in a block, the hash of that block will change, breaking the chain and alerting the network to the tampering. This immutability ensures that medical data stored on a blockchain is trustworthy and cannot be tampered with after it has been recorded. For healthcare providers, this means that patient records, clinical trial data, and other sensitive information can be relied upon as accurate and unaltered.
- *Encryption and Privacy*: Blockchain uses advanced cryptographic techniques to secure data. Each transaction on a blockchain is encrypted using public and private keys, ensuring that only authorized parties can access the information. Public keys act as digital addresses on the blockchain, while private keys are used to sign transactions and verify ownership of data [17]. This encryption ensures that patient data remains private and secure, even in a decentralized network. Additionally, blockchain can support privacy-preserving technologies, such as zero-knowledge proofs, which allow transactions to be verified without revealing the underlying data.
- *Consensus Mechanisms*: Blockchain networks use consensus mechanisms to validate transactions and ensure the integrity of the data recorded on the blockchain. Common consensus mechanisms include PoW and PoS, which require network participants to agree on the validity of transactions before they are added to the blockchain. These mechanisms prevent unauthorized transactions and ensure that all participants in the network adhere to the same set of rules. In healthcare, consensus mechanisms can help ensure that only verified and authorized data is added to the blockchain, further enhancing the security and integrity of medical records.
- *Reduced Attack Surface*: In a centralized system, the entire database is stored in a single location, making it an attractive target for hackers. If an attacker breaches the central server, they can potentially gain access to the entire dataset. Blockchain, on the other hand, distributes data across multiple nodes, reducing the attack surface and making it more difficult for hackers to compromise the system. Even if an attacker were to gain control of a few nodes, they would not be able to alter the data on the blockchain without the consensus of the majority of the network. This distributed security model makes blockchain a more secure option for storing sensitive medical information.
- *Smart Contracts for Automated Security and Compliance*: Smart contracts, which are self-executing contracts with the terms of the agreement written directly into code, can further enhance security in blockchain-based healthcare systems. Smart contracts can automate security protocols, such as access controls and data-sharing permissions, ensuring that only authorized parties can access specific data. They can also enforce compliance with regulatory requirements, such as HIPAA or GDPR,

by automatically auditing transactions and ensuring that data is handled according to the rules. This automation reduces the risk of human error and ensures that security and compliance protocols are consistently followed.

7.10 TRANSPARENCY: ENHANCING TRUST AND ACCOUNTABILITY

Transparency is another significant advantage of blockchain technology, particularly in industries where trust and accountability are critical. In healthcare, transparency can help build trust between patients, providers, and other stakeholders by ensuring that data handling practices are visible, auditable, and compliant with ethical and regulatory standards. Blockchain's transparent nature can address several key challenges in medical data management, including data provenance, auditability, and accountability.

- *Data Provenance and Traceability*: Blockchain's transparent ledger allows for the complete traceability of data from its origin to its current state. Each transaction on the blockchain is recorded with a timestamp and linked to the previous transaction, creating an unbroken chain of custody for the data. In healthcare, this transparency can be used to track the provenance of medical records, ensuring that healthcare providers can verify the source and history of the data. For example, blockchain can help trace the lifecycle of a patient's medical record, from initial diagnosis to subsequent treatments and follow-up care. This traceability can also be applied to medical research, where blockchain can be used to track the origins and integrity of clinical trial data, ensuring that the results are accurate and reliable.
- *Auditability and Regulatory Compliance*: Blockchain's transparent and immutable ledger provides a built-in audit trail that can be used to verify compliance with regulatory requirements. In traditional systems, audits often require manual reviews of data and processes, which can be time-consuming and prone to errors. Blockchain automates the audit process by providing a complete and verifiable record of all transactions. This auditability ensures that healthcare organizations can demonstrate compliance with regulations such as HIPAA, GDPR, and other data protection laws [18]. For example, blockchain can be used to track access to patient records, ensuring that only authorized individuals have viewed or modified the data. This level of transparency can help healthcare organizations avoid costly fines and legal penalties for non-compliance.
- *Accountability and Trust*: Transparency is essential for building trust in the healthcare system, particularly when it comes to the handling of sensitive patient information. Blockchain's transparent ledger ensures that all transactions are visible to authorized participants in the network, creating a system of accountability. In a blockchain-based healthcare system, patients can see who has accessed their medical records and for what purpose, giving them greater confidence that their data is being handled responsibly [18]. This transparency can also help build trust between healthcare

providers and patients, as providers can demonstrate that they are following best practices for data security and privacy.

- *Enabling Ethical Data Sharing*: Blockchain's transparency can also facilitate ethical data-sharing practices in healthcare. One of the challenges in medical data management is balancing the need for data sharing (e.g., for research or public health purposes) with the need to protect patient privacy. Blockchain can enable secure and transparent data sharing by allowing patients to grant specific permissions for the use of their data while ensuring that all transactions are recorded and auditable. For example, patients can use blockchain to consent to the sharing of their anonymized data for medical research, with the assurance that their privacy will be protected and that their data will be used ethically [19].

In addition to ensuring integrity, blockchain also enhances data accessibility. By providing a decentralized network, blockchain allows authorized parties to access data in real time from anywhere in the world. This has significant implications for patient care, particularly in emergency situations where timely access to medical records can be life-saving. Moreover, blockchain's transparency allows patients to have greater control over their data. They can grant or revoke access to their medical information, ensuring that their privacy is respected.

7.11 USE CASES OF BLOCKCHAIN IN MEDICAL DATA MANAGEMENT

Blockchain technology can revolutionize the way medical data is managed by providing innovative solutions to various challenges in healthcare. Below are several use cases where blockchain can be effectively applied in medical data management:

- *EHRs Management*:
  - Blockchain can create a decentralized system for storing and sharing EHRs across different healthcare providers.
  - Patients can grant and revoke access to their records using cryptographic keys, ensuring privacy and control over their health data.
  - Interoperability issues between different EHR systems can be resolved, enabling seamless data exchange across the healthcare ecosystem.
- *Patient Data Security and Privacy*:
  - Blockchain's cryptographic features can protect sensitive patient information from unauthorized access and cyberattacks.
  - Data stored on the blockchain is immutable, meaning that once it is recorded, it cannot be altered or deleted without detection.
  - Patients can control who has access to their data, improving trust and transparency in healthcare services.
- *Clinical Trials and Research Data Management*:
  - Blockchain can be used to ensure the integrity and transparency of clinical trial data by creating an immutable record of trial results.

    - Researchers can track and verify the origin of data, ensuring the validity of research findings.
    - Blockchain can also be used to facilitate the secure sharing of anonymized patient data for research purposes while ensuring compliance with privacy regulations.
- *Supply Chain Management for Pharmaceuticals*:
    - Blockchain can track the entire supply chain of pharmaceuticals, from manufacturing to distribution, ensuring that medications are authentic and have not been tampered with.
    - This helps in combating counterfeit drugs, which are a significant global issue, and ensures that patients receive genuine medications.
    - Blockchain can also track expiration dates, recalls, and other important information related to pharmaceutical products.
- *Consent Management*:
    - Blockchain can provide a secure and transparent system for managing patient consent for data sharing and medical procedures.
    - Patients can provide consent digitally through smart contracts, which automatically enforce consent terms and conditions.
    - The blockchain ledger keeps a permanent record of consent agreements, which can be audited at any time to ensure compliance with legal and ethical standards.
- *Insurance Claims Processing*:
    - Blockchain can streamline the insurance claims process by providing a transparent and tamper-proof record of medical treatments and procedures.
    - Smart contracts can automate the claims approval process, reducing administrative overhead and preventing fraud.
    - Insurance companies can verify the authenticity of claims in real time, leading to faster reimbursements for patients and healthcare providers.
- *Telemedicine and Remote Monitoring*:
    - Blockchain can securely store and transmit data generated by telemedicine consultations and remote monitoring devices, ensuring that this data is accurate and tamper-proof.
    - Patients can grant temporary access to their health data to remote healthcare providers, ensuring continuity of care across different platforms.
    - Blockchain can also be used to create a unified patient profile that integrates data from various sources, such as wearable devices, ensuring comprehensive and personalized care.
- *Medical Credentialing and Licensing*:
    - Blockchain can be used to create a verifiable record of healthcare professionals' credentials, licenses, and certifications.
    - This ensures that only qualified professionals are allowed to practice, reducing the risk of fraud and improving patient safety.

  - Credentialing data on the blockchain is immutable and easily accessible, streamlining the verification process for hospitals, clinics, and other healthcare institutions.
- *Genomic Data Management*:
  - Blockchain can provide a secure platform for storing and sharing genomic data, ensuring that this highly sensitive information is protected from unauthorized access.
  - Patients can control how their genomic data is used, whether for research, personalized medicine, or other purposes, by granting permissions through blockchain.
  - Researchers can also benefit from blockchain's transparency, ensuring that genomic data is accurate and traceable to its original source.
- *Public Health and Epidemiology*:
  - Blockchain can be used to securely aggregate and analyze health data for public health initiatives, such as tracking the spread of infectious diseases.
  - Public health agencies can use blockchain to share data across different regions and organizations, ensuring timely and accurate responses to health crises.
  - Blockchain's transparency ensures that public health data is reliable and can be audited by authorized entities, improving trust in the data.
- *Personal Health Records (PHR)*:
  - Blockchain can enable patients to manage their own health records, consolidating data from multiple sources such as hospitals, labs, and wearable devices into a single, secure record.
  - Patients can share their personal health records with healthcare providers as needed, ensuring continuity of care across different facilities and treatments.
  - Blockchain ensures that PHR data remains private and secure, giving patients full control over who has access to their information.

These use cases demonstrate the transformative potential of blockchain in medical data management. By enhancing security, transparency, and interoperability, blockchain can address many of the challenges faced by the healthcare industry, ultimately leading to better patient outcomes and more efficient healthcare delivery.

7.12 ADDRESSING CHALLENGES IN BLOCKCHAIN ADOPTION

While blockchain technology holds significant promise for transforming medical data management, its adoption in healthcare faces several challenges. Addressing these challenges is crucial for successful implementation [19]. Below are key challenges and potential solutions presented in Table 7.1 for clarity.

By addressing the challenges presented in Table 7.1, healthcare organizations can more effectively harness the potential of blockchain technology to transform medical data management, enhance patient care, and ensure the security and integrity of health information.

TABLE 7.1
Challenges and Solutions in Blockchain Adoption for Medical Data Management [19]

Challenge	Description	Solution
Scalability	Blockchain networks may struggle with handling large volumes of transactions.	Implement layer-2 solutions, permissioned blockchains, and hybrid models with off-chain storage.
Data Privacy and Security	Storing sensitive medical data on blockchain raises privacy concerns.	Use cryptographic techniques, off-chain storage, and permissioned blockchains to enhance privacy and security.
Regulatory Compliance	Blockchain must comply with healthcare regulations (e.g., HIPAA, GDPR).	Collaborate with regulators, use smart contracts for compliance, and conduct regular audits.
Interoperability	Lack of standardization and compatibility between blockchain platforms.	Develop standardized protocols, support cross-chain technologies, and advocate for industry-wide standards.
High Energy Consumption	Proof of Work (PoW) blockchains are energy-intensive.	Transition to energy-efficient consensus mechanisms (e.g., PoS, PoA) and use permissioned blockchains.
Cost of Implementation	High initial costs of implementing blockchain in healthcare systems.	Start with pilot projects, leverage blockchain-as-a-service (BaaS), and form partnerships to reduce costs.
Legal and Ethical Issues	Legal and ethical challenges, such as determining liability and consent.	Develop legal frameworks, ensure consent mechanisms, and collaborate with legal and ethical experts.
User Adoption and Education	Resistance from healthcare providers and patients due to lack of understanding.	Provide education and training, develop user-friendly applications, and engage stakeholders early to build trust.

7.13 THE ROLE OF SMART CONTRACTS IN HEALTHCARE AUTOMATION

Smart contracts are self-executing contracts with the terms of the agreement directly written into code. In healthcare, they play a crucial role in automating various processes, improving efficiency, reducing costs, and ensuring transparency [20–22]. Following (Figure 7.3) are key roles that smart contracts can play in healthcare automation.

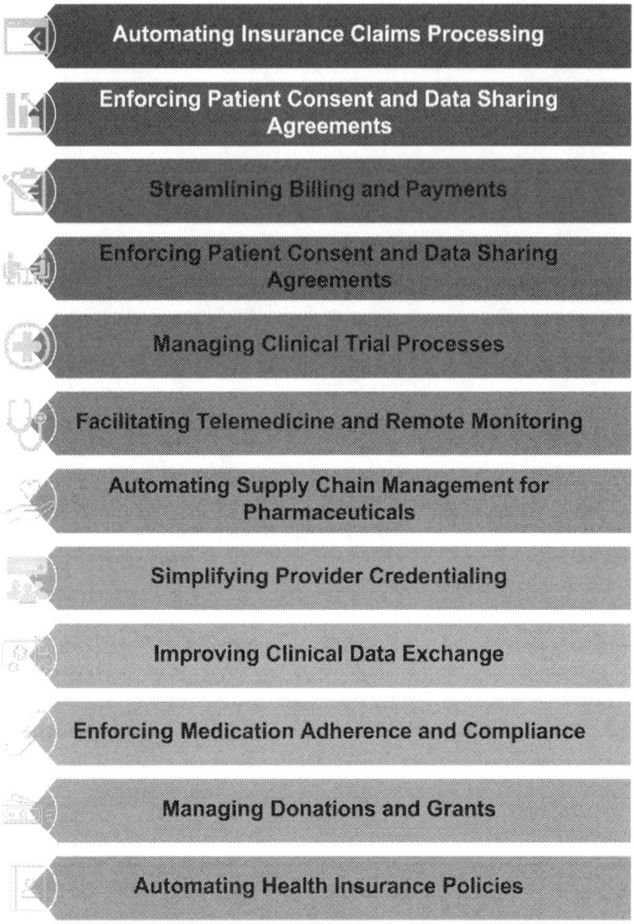

FIGURE 7.3 Roles of smart contracts in healthcare automation.

- *Automating Insurance Claims Processing*:
  - Smart contracts can automatically verify insurance claims, check policy coverage, and execute payments when conditions are met, reducing manual processing time and errors.
  - They help in preventing fraud by verifying treatment records and insurance details on a decentralized ledger.
  - Patients and providers benefit from faster claim settlements, improving patient satisfaction and provider revenue cycles.
- *Streamlining Billing and Payments*:
  - Smart contracts can automate healthcare billing by generating invoices and facilitating direct payments between patients, providers, and insurers.

    - They can eliminate intermediaries, reducing administrative costs and delays in payment processing.
    - The transparency of smart contracts ensures that billing discrepancies and disputes are minimized, leading to smoother financial transactions.
- *Enforcing Patient Consent and Data-Sharing Agreements*:
    - Smart contracts can manage patient consent for data sharing, ensuring that data is only shared with authorized parties and under agreed conditions.
    - They allow patients to revoke or modify consent at any time, automatically updating access rights across the network.
    - This increases patient control over their medical data while ensuring compliance with data protection regulations.
- *Managing Clinical Trial Processes*:
    - Smart contracts can automate various aspects of clinical trials, such as patient enrollment, randomization, and tracking of participation.
    - They can ensure that trial data is collected, verified, and shared in compliance with regulatory requirements, improving transparency and trust.
    - Payments to participants, researchers, and institutions can be automated, ensuring timely compensation and reducing administrative overhead.
- *Facilitating Telemedicine and Remote Monitoring*:
    - Smart contracts can automate the scheduling, billing, and data transfer processes in telemedicine, ensuring that healthcare providers are compensated based on pre-set agreements.
    - They can also automatically trigger alerts or notifications if remote monitoring data, such as vital signs, exceeds predefined thresholds, initiating a real-time response from healthcare providers.
    - This ensures timely and efficient care for patients, especially those in remote or underserved areas.
- *Automating Supply Chain Management for Pharmaceuticals*:
    - Smart contracts can track and verify the entire lifecycle of pharmaceutical products, from manufacturing to distribution to end-users, ensuring authenticity and compliance with regulatory standards.
    - They can automatically trigger payments at different stages of the supply chain once specific conditions, such as delivery verification, are met.
    - The automation reduces paperwork, enhances transparency, and combats the issue of counterfeit drugs in the market.
- *Simplifying Provider Credentialing*:
    - Smart contracts can automate the credentialing process for healthcare providers, verifying their qualifications, certifications, and licenses in real time.
    - This reduces the time and cost associated with manual credentialing, ensuring that qualified professionals can begin practicing sooner.

    - The use of blockchain for storing credentialing information ensures that the data is secure, tamper-proof, and easily accessible by authorized parties.
- *Improving Clinical Data Exchange:*
    - Smart contracts can govern the exchange of clinical data between different healthcare providers, ensuring that data is shared securely and in compliance with regulations.
    - They can automatically execute data-sharing agreements, granting access to relevant parties and revoking access when no longer necessary.
    - This enhances interoperability and ensures that patient data is available when and where it is needed for treatment.
- *Enforcing Medication Adherence and Compliance*:
    - Smart contracts can be integrated with IoT devices or mobile health apps to monitor patient adherence to prescribed medication regimens.
    - They can trigger reminders or notifications if a patient misses a dose, and automatically notify healthcare providers if there is a pattern of non-adherence.
    - This automation helps in ensuring that patients follow their treatment plans, leading to better health outcomes.
- *Managing Donations and Grants*:
    - Smart contracts can automate the disbursement of funds from donations and grants, ensuring that the money is released only when specific conditions are met, such as the completion of a research milestone or delivery of healthcare services.
    - This ensures transparency and accountability in the use of funds, reducing the potential for misuse and ensuring that the intended recipients benefit.
- *Automating Health Insurance Policies*:
    - Smart contracts can be used to create and manage health insurance policies, automatically adjusting coverage based on changes in the policyholder's health or other conditions.
    - They can automatically enforce policy terms, such as co-pays, deductibles, and exclusions, ensuring that all parties adhere to the agreed conditions.
    - The automation reduces administrative overhead and ensures that both patients and insurers have a clear understanding of their obligations.

7.13.1 Case Studies: Real-World Applications of Blockchain in Medical Data Management

Blockchain technology is increasingly being adopted across the healthcare industry to address the challenges of medical data management. Below are detailed case studies that showcase real-world applications of blockchain in various aspects of healthcare, demonstrating the transformative potential of this technology.

MEDREC: A BLOCKCHAIN-BASED EHR SYSTEM

BACKGROUND

MedRec is an Ethereum-based blockchain platform developed by MIT Media Lab in collaboration with Beth Israel Deaconess Medical Center. The platform is designed to improve the management of EHRs by ensuring data integrity, security, and patient ownership [21, 22].

APPLICATION

- *Decentralized Data Storage*: MedRec uses a blockchain to store patient metadata, while the actual medical data remains in the providers' databases. This ensures that the data remains decentralized, and no single entity has full control over it.
- *Patient-Centric Control*: Patients have full control over their medical records, deciding who can access their data and for how long. They can easily revoke access when necessary, thus enhancing privacy and data security.
- *Interoperability*: MedRec bridges the gap between different healthcare systems by enabling seamless data exchange across different EHR systems, thus addressing interoperability challenges.

OUTCOMES

- *Data Security and Integrity*: The blockchain ensures that medical data is tamper-proof, reducing the risk of data breaches and ensuring the integrity of medical records.
- *Improved Patient Engagement*: By giving patients control over their health data, MedRec fosters greater patient engagement in their healthcare journey.
- *Interoperability Enhancement*: MedRec's architecture allows for interoperability between disparate healthcare systems, ensuring continuity of care across multiple providers.

CHALLENGES

- *Scalability Issues*: Like many blockchain applications, MedRec faces scalability challenges, especially as the volume of healthcare data continues to grow.
- *Adoption Barriers*: Widespread adoption requires integration with existing EHR systems, which can be complex and costly for healthcare providers.

GUARD TIME: SECURING ESTONIA'S NATIONAL HEALTH SYSTEM

BACKGROUND

Estonia, known for its advanced digital infrastructure, implemented blockchain technology in its national healthcare system in partnership with guard time, a blockchain-based cybersecurity company [21, 22]. The goal was to enhance the security and integrity of medical records for all Estonian citizens.

APPLICATION

- *Immutable Audit Trails*: Guard time's blockchain solution creates immutable audit trails for all medical records. This ensures that any access, modification, or sharing of medical data is recorded and cannot be altered or deleted, providing transparency and accountability.
- *Data Integrity*: The blockchain verifies the integrity of medical records by creating cryptographic signatures for each piece of data. Any attempt to tamper with the data can be detected immediately, ensuring the authenticity of the information.
- *Automated Verification*: Healthcare providers, insurers, and other authorized parties can automatically verify the integrity of medical records without relying on centralized databases or intermediaries.

OUTCOMES

- *Enhanced Security*: Guard time's blockchain implementation has significantly reduced the risk of data breaches and cyberattacks on Estonia's healthcare system.
- *Trust and Transparency*: The immutable audit trails have enhanced trust between patients, healthcare providers, and government agencies, as all interactions with medical data are transparent and verifiable.
- *Regulatory Compliance*: The blockchain-based system helps Estonia comply with data protection regulations such as the GDPR, as it provides secure and auditable records of data access and sharing.

CHALLENGES

- *Complexity of Integration*: Integrating blockchain into a national healthcare system requires significant effort and collaboration between different stakeholders, including government agencies, healthcare providers, and technology experts.
- *Initial Costs*: The initial implementation of the blockchain system was costly, but the long-term benefits in terms of security and efficiency are expected to outweigh these costs.

BURSTIQ: EMPOWERING PERSONAL HEALTH MANAGEMENT WITH BLOCKCHAIN

BACKGROUND

BurstIQ is a blockchain-based platform that focuses on personal health management, enabling patients to own and control their health data. The platform aims to create a health data marketplace where individuals can securely share their data with healthcare providers, researchers, and insurers.

APPLICATION

- *Personal Health Wallet*: BurstIQ provides patients with a "Health Wallet" that stores their medical records, genetic information, and lifestyle data. Patients can choose to share specific pieces of data with healthcare providers, insurers, or researchers, ensuring privacy and control.
- *Data Monetization*: Patients can monetize their health data by sharing it with researchers or companies conducting clinical trials. The blockchain ensures that patients receive compensation for their data, and they can track how their data is used.
- *Interoperability and Accessibility*: BurstIQ's platform connects various data sources, including EHR systems, wearable devices, and genomic data, creating a unified health record that patients can access and manage.

OUTCOMES

- *Empowered Patients*: BurstIQ's platform gives patients unprecedented control over their health data, allowing them to manage their PHI and share it as they see fit.
- *Data-Driven Insights*: By aggregating data from various sources, BurstIQ enables healthcare providers to gain deeper insights into a patient's health, leading to more personalized and effective care.
- *New Revenue Streams*: The ability to monetize health data creates new revenue streams for patients, particularly those who participate in research studies or clinical trials.

CHALLENGES

- *Data Privacy Concerns*: Although blockchain enhances security, some patients may still have concerns about sharing their health data, especially with commercial entities.
- *Regulatory Hurdles*: BurstIQ must navigate complex regulatory landscapes, ensuring that its data-sharing marketplace complies with privacy laws and regulations.

7.14 THE FUTURE OF BLOCKCHAIN IN HEALTHCARE

The future of blockchain in healthcare is promising, with many potential applications yet to be fully explored. As the technology continues to evolve, we can expect to see more widespread adoption of blockchain for medical data management. Advances in scaling solutions, improved interoperability, and the development of standardized protocols will further enhance the effectiveness of blockchain in healthcare.

Moreover, as patient demand for greater control over their data grows, blockchain may play a central role in creating patient-centered healthcare systems. By empowering patients with control over their data, blockchain has the potential to shift the balance of power in healthcare, fostering a more transparent, secure, and equitable system. Table 7.2 presents a tabular form of the future of blockchain in healthcare.

TABLE 7.2
Future of Blockchain in Healthcare [22]

Area of Impact	Future Developments	Expected Benefits	Challenges
Patient-centric healthcare	Patient ownership of health data Personalized care Data portability	Increased patient autonomy, improved collaboration, access to comprehensive health records	Patient engagement • Technology integration
Data interoperability	• Universal health records • Standardized data protocols • Interoperable networks	• Seamless data exchange • Continuity of care • Reduced fragmentation of health data	Creating interoperability standards • Cross-chain integration
Data security and privacy	• Immutable records • Advanced encryption techniques • Decentralized identity management	• Enhanced data privacy • Protection against tampering • Reduced risk of identity theft	Regulatory compliance • Managing decentralized identities
Clinical research and trials	Transparent and tamper-proof data • Automated consent management • Incentivized participation	• Increased trust in research • Faster research cycles • Broader participation	Ethical and legal considerations • Gaining patient trust
Supply chain management	• End-to-end traceability • Automated compliance with regulations • Real-time monitoring	• Reduced counterfeit drugs • Increased transparency • Improved supply chain efficiency	• Industry-wide collaboration • Legacy system integration
Health insurance models	• Smart insurance contracts • Fraud reduction • Peer-to-peer (P2P) insurance models	• Automated claims processing • Reduced fraud • Affordable alternatives to traditional insurance models	• Regulatory challenges • Technology adoption barriers

(Continued)

TABLE 7.2 ***(Continued)***
Future of Blockchain in Healthcare [22]

Area of Impact	Future Developments	Expected Benefits	Challenges
Blockchain and AI integration	• AI-driven insights on blockchain • Decentralized AI models • Automated decision-making	Data security and AI synergy • More accurate AI models • Transparent AI-driven decisions	Ensuring AI fairness • Data-sharing limitations
Policy and regulatory evolution	• Blockchain-specific regulations • Global collaboration • Ethical guidelines	• Clearer legal frameworks • Increased adoption and innovation • Responsible blockchain usage	• Developing adaptive policies • Global standardization

7.15 CONCLUSION

Blockchain technology has immense potential to revolutionize healthcare by transforming the way medical data is managed, stored, and accessed. With its decentralized, secure, and transparent nature, blockchain can address many of the longstanding challenges in the healthcare industry, such as data silos, privacy concerns, and inefficiencies in the supply chain.

By empowering patients with greater control over their health data, improving interoperability between different healthcare systems, and strengthening data security, blockchain can enable more patient-centric and efficient healthcare delivery. The integration of blockchain with emerging technologies like AI and smart contracts further amplifies its potential, opening new possibilities for automation, personalized care, and real-time decision-making. However, the road to widespread blockchain adoption in healthcare is not without challenges. Issues such as regulatory compliance, standardization, and industry-wide collaboration must be addressed to ensure that blockchain-based solutions are implemented effectively and responsibly. Policymakers, technologists, and healthcare providers must work together to create a framework that balances innovation with ethical considerations and patient rights.

In the future, as blockchain technology continues to mature and become more integrated into healthcare systems, it is poised to play a pivotal role in creating a more transparent, secure, and equitable healthcare environment. The continued evolution of blockchain in healthcare will ultimately lead to better outcomes for patients, providers, and the entire healthcare ecosystem.

REFERENCES

1. K. Park and M. Y. Chung, "A Study on Healthcare Big Data Management System using Distributed File System," IEEE Access, vol. 6, pp. 66187–66195, 2018.
2. S. Grigorescu, A. M. Grigorescu, and I. Antonya, "Medical Big Data and Deep Learning Techniques: Opportunities and Challenges," in Proc. IEEE Int. Conf. Systems, Man, and Cybernetics (SMC), Miyazaki, Japan, 2018, pp. 1000–1005.

3. P. Kuniyal, A. Singh, and A. Bhatt, "Detection Techniques Used For Foodborne Pathogens and Its Significant Financial and Human Behavioral Effects," JRTDD, vol. 6, no. 2s, pp. 181–184, Mar. 2023.
4. L. A. Gordon and T. Loeb, "The Economics of Information Security Investment," ACM Transactions on Information and System Security (TISSEC), vol. 5, no. 4, pp. 438–457, Nov. 2002.
5. A. B. Hamadeh, R. E. Malas, M. N. Alhamid, and S. A. Almalki, "A Survey on Big Data Cloud Computing Security: The Healthcare Case," IEEE Access, vol. 8, pp. 29767–29791, 2020.
6. M. Saleh, S. Darwish, and R. Potluri, "Security and Privacy Concerns in Big Data Health Care," IEEE Access, vol. 7, pp. 532–546, 2019.
7. P. Kumar, R. Chaudhary, A. Aggarwal, P. Singh, and R. Tomar. "Improving Medical Image Segmentation Techniques Using Multiphase Level Set Approach Via Bias Correction." (2012).
8. H. J. Park and B. Lee, "Big Data and Healthcare: Theoretical Framework and Big Data Application in Medicine and Healthcare," Journal of Biosciences and Medicines, vol. 5, no. 11, pp. 10–15, Nov. 2017.
9. J. Tang, J. Ren, and M. Wu, "Research on Medical Data Interoperability," in Proc. IEEE Int. Conf. e-Health Networking, Applications and Services (HealthCom), Lyon, France, 2016, pp. 1–6.
10. A. Bhatt, P. Joshi, and G. Aggarwal, "Smart Blind Stick Data Logging: Enhancing Safety and Accessibility," in 2024 International Conference on Healthcare Innovations, Software and Engineering Technologies (HISET), Jan. 2024, pp. 176–180.
11. A. T. Rashid and T. M. Rahman, "Improving Data Interoperability in Healthcare Systems Using Ontologies," in Proc. IEEE Int. Conf. Bioinformatics and Biomedicine (BIBM), Philadelphia, PA, 2016, pp. 1052–1059.
12. F. F. Suleiman, M. L. Lamoureux, and B. W. Surgenor, "Privacy-Preserving Data Analytics for Healthcare: A Blockchain-Based Framework," in Proc. IEEE Int. Conf. Systems, Man, and Cybernetics (SMC), Toronto, ON, 2020, pp. 2132–2139.
13. N. Kshetri, "Blockchain's Roles in Strengthening Cybersecurity and Protecting Privacy," Telecommunications Policy, vol. 41, no. 10, pp. 1027–1038, Nov. 2017.
14. A. Abouelmehdi, A. Beni-Hessane, and H. Khaloufi, "Big Healthcare Data: Preserving Security and Privacy," Journal of Big Data, vol. 5, no. 1, pp. 1–18, Dec. 2018.
15. P. Sharma, M. D. Borah, and S. Namasudra, "Improving security of medical big data by using Blockchain technology," Computers and Electrical Engineering, vol. 96, pp. 107529.
16. A. Miller and J. Pagliery, "Health Care Data Security: Current Practices and Trends in Data Breach Prevention," Health Policy and Technology, vol. 9, no. 2, pp. 207–215, June 2020.
17. O. Arshi, G. Gupta, and A. Aggarwal, "IoT Forensics," in Advanced Techniques and Applications of Cybersecurity and Forensics, 1st ed., Boca Raton, FL: Chapman and Hall/CRC, 2024, pp. 57–81.
18. S. R. Chowdhury et al., "Challenges in the Era of Big Data for Healthcare: Multi-Omics Data Integration and AI Technologies," IEEE Reviews in Biomedical Engineering, vol. 13, pp. 227–246, 2020.
19. T. R. Frieden, "Data Modernization and Interoperability in Public Health: Progress, Challenges, and Opportunities," The Lancet Public Health, vol. 6, no. 7, pp. 469–477, Jul. 2021.
20. A. Bonner, "Data Security in Health Care: The Impact of Cybersecurity Breaches and How to Prevent Them," Journal of Medical Systems, vol. 44, no. 1, pp. 1–15, Jan. 2020.
21. D. McCoy, and T. S. Sharma, "The Future of Medical Data Management: Regulatory, Technical, and Ethical Challenges," Journal of Medical Internet Research, vol. 22, no. 11, pp. 23–34, Nov. 2020.
22. C. S. Kruse et al., "Challenges in Healthcare Data Management and Research: Big Data Privacy and Ethical Considerations," BMC Health Services Research, vol. 18, no. 1, pp. 1–9, Dec. 2018.

8 Exploring the Role of Steganography in Securing Healthcare Data

Deeya Rajput, Dhruv Sharma, and Rohit Tanwar

8.1 INTRODUCTION

The mechanism that provides safe communication wherein all the critical information is hidden in seemingly innocent carriers, such as text, audio, or graphics, is known as steganography. Protection systems like this are definitely essential in the healthcare setting, considering that medical records comprise confidential personal and clinical information. The risk factors associated with data breaches and illegal access increase because of the increase in the use of electronic health information systems. This increases the strength of healthcare data security by enciphering sensitive information, such as patient records or private communications, inside such digital media. Besides preventing the possibility of data breaches, this approach preserves the confidentiality and confidence of patients—two factors germane to the integrity of healthcare systems.

In the healthcare sector, steganography becomes particularly significant due to the sensitive nature of medical records. Electronic health records (EHRs) contain highly sensitive data, such as patient medical histories, diagnoses, treatment plans, and personal identification information. The confidentiality of this data is paramount to avoid misuse, fraud, and to maintain patient trust [1]. Data breaches in healthcare can lead to serious consequences, including compromised patient safety, identity theft, and significant financial losses for healthcare providers [2].

Healthcare entities, therefore, need strong measures to protect this information. Apart from their encrypted nature, steganography provides yet another level of ensuring the data is hidden by keeping the sensitive info away within digital files. Combined with encryption, this shielding makes the data even more difficult to locate and retrieve by outside actors [3]. For the purposes of exchanging and broadcasting medical images, this can be a very useful scenario to protect the patient's privacy without sacrificing image utility for diagnosis by hiding sensitive information directly into images.

Healthcare data is being seriously threatened not only because of the financial loss but also because it severely damaged their reputation and patient trust. By imbedding steganography this risk is minimized as only part of the data just

DOI: 10.1201/9781003510932-8

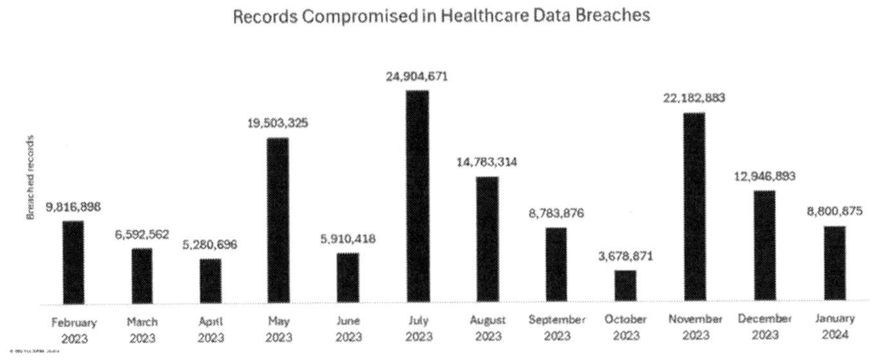

FIGURE 8.1 Healthcare data breach statistics [5].

visible, bringing about that if someone were to hack into health chambers records, by steganography they could be prevented from nibbling at the most sensitive bits of information which remains hidden in plain view. Combining steganography with conventional healthcare data security frameworks, institutions can reinforce their access protection and cyber safety [4]. Figure 8.1 shows the record of healthcare breaches till January 2024.

Healthcare information envelops a wide cluster of delicate data, counting therapeutic histories, analysis, medications, individual data, and protection points of interest [6]. As EHRs, medical imaging systems, and telemedicine platforms integrate more deeply into healthcare, ensuring the privacy, availability, and integrity of this data becomes critical [7]. This data is highly valued on the dark web, making it an attractive target for fraudsters for identity theft and insurance fraud [8].

Steganography has many applications and advantages over protecting the data of healthcare. It ensures the embedding of sensitive information inside digital images or audio files or video streams in a way that remains imperceptible to the naked eye, thus securing data from interceptors while not disturbing the usability of the steganographic medium [9, 10]. Example: Patient identifiers or diagnostic codes can be hidden into the pixel values of medical images in a way that does not affect their diagnostic quality using Least Significant Bit (LSB) embedding [10]. This is very useful in ensuring confidentiality for EHRs and other sensitive data in healthcare, as even if unauthorized people get hold of the files, they cannot not retrieve the information that was embedded [9, 10].

Use of steganography, in concert with improved authentication, encryption, and strong access controls, tends to reduce the threat of a data breach and strengthens general data security in healthcare systems [10]. The new generation steganographic techniques that are emerging based on Machine Learning (ML) and Artificial Intelligence (AI) have opened new avenues both for embedding data and for resistance to detection [10]. Future developments along these lines will thus cement the growth of the concept, focusing more on the importance of steganography as a constituent part of a data security framework for healthcare [11].

It is, therefore, with the help of such a multilayered security framework, which includes checks on data integrity, encryption, steganography, as well as access controls that may be able to offer the needed protection against exposure of clinical data [12]. Encryption serves to protect data by read making it unintelligible in case intercepted; where access control will ensure that only those who are duly authorized unlock important securing doors, which will include things such as role-based access or multi-factor authentication.

To truly safeguard healthcare information, there is a need for the implementation of a multilayered security stack that includes data integrity, encryption, steganography as well as access control mechanisms [12]. The purpose of encryption is to make sure that the information that has been intercepted cannot be understood without the appropriate key, while access control policies such as role-based access and two-factor authentication ensure that only permitted staff have access. This is also assisted by steganography, which is the technique of hiding data inside non-sensitive data, like embedding fingerprints inside images of files. Regular assessments and active post-deployment assessments are necessary in order to discover weaknesses and to comply with the rules.

The benefits of steganography over other techniques for securing data are that the secret information can be placed imperceptibly inside other multimedia data, and this is why it is considered more desirable compared to healthcare data security [13]. For instance, LSB embedding techniques can conceal patient information in the LSBs of the pixels in medical images but do not detract from the diagnostic utility of the images. This method is applicable as well to biological signals such as ECG waveforms, which inherently may carry steganographically encoded patient information without impairment of their diagnostic utility [14]. Steganography, applied with cryptographic mechanisms provides additional strength to protection. Even if data is detected as being hidden, it is still protected because of the encryption.

Despite its promising nature, just like many encryption techniques, steganography has a few limitations to healthcare data security. Computational overhead and storage are the main constraints that have prevented applications due to slow systems from hiding and extracting the hidden data in large files such as images. A further limitation is the balance between data embedding capacity and preserving the quality of the original file; hence, its applicability practically has been its limitation. Another threat is emerging in this ever-evolving field of steganalysis; therefore, constant development of steganographic methods should remain up to date [15]. Trying to abide by regulatory standards for healthcare such as HIPAA and GDPR, steganography exacerbates challenges in deployment-frequently demanding legal access to data and a method for auditability.

The future directions of healthcare steganography try to increase the capacity of embedding the data, reduce the computational overhead, and optimize the efficiency of the algorithm. Some new approaches, DNA-based and neural network-based steganography may bypass the existing problems associated with this field [16]. Steganography combined with ML improves data embedding techniques, and detection, and prevents malicious access to the content. Real-time data embedding and extraction technologies can hasten the safe transfer of sensitive patient information, hence highly benefiting healthcare delivery [16]. The development of steganalysis-resistant systems is crucial to ensure that healthcare data remains resilient and confidential with a sophisticated detection technique in place [16].

As the healthcare sector becomes more technologically inclined, the safeguarding of sensitive patient information becomes ever more critical. Even though such procedures as encryption are of extreme relevance, they may work out to be insufficient whenever the threats are sophisticated attacks. This helps in heightening the advantage of steganography as it conceals and embeds messages within a cover medium that is not suspected by intruders as containing such sensitive information [16]. With some modifications—namely embedding steganography into the healthcare security policies and procedures along with the encryption and access control technologies—healthcare organizations are better positioned to protect their patient data against privacy and security breaches [17]. So far, the widespread adoption of steganography and its further development invites optimism for the improvement of the reliability of safety and expediency of healthcare data in a networked world [16].

8.2 LITERATURE REVIEW

It comes from the Greek words "steganos" meaning covered and "graphein" meaning writing. Steganography thus refers to the act of concealing information within other, not-sensitive media such that it becomes invisible or hidden from unauthorized users. It's crucial in the healthcare industry in this stage of change toward digitalization with the rising requirement of securing electronically transmitted and stored sensitive data, comprising personal information, diagnostic imagery, and medical records.

Data security within the healthcare domain is quite crucial as medical records are sensitive information that has to be shared extensively over public networks very often. While traditional cryptographic methods do mask data quite well, they do not camouflage the very fact of the presence of data, and they may still attract unwanted eyes and potential breaches. Steganography, on the other hand, conceals the existence of secret information within innocuous text audio or image files [18]. This gives a dual layer of security in the encryption-steganography layer. Here, if someone suspects that some data might be embedded somewhere, they will not be able to retrieve that information without the appropriate decryption keys.

Very important in the medical diagnosis and treatment phases, the digital images from CT, MRI, and X-ray scans represent very high-resolution and complex structures. Therefore, they offer an excellent carrier for hidden data without degrading diagnostic quality [19, 20]. Sensitive information such as diagnoses, plans of treatment, or clinical history may be hidden within these images; therefore, even if intercepted, the secret data remains intact.

Steganography is a technique that conceals data within other non-sensitive media. This technique is not confined to digital images only; it can be implemented in many other domains apart from digital images. In the health sector, the need to securely and discreetly store data is greatly in demand because medical information is highly sensitive. The flexibility of the technique allows its implementation over various media forms, therefore improving the security and confidentiality of data in many contexts. Below, we elaborate on the mechanisms and benefits of text, audio, and hybrid systems in healthcare using steganography.

Image steganography is the technique by which sensitive information, such as patient data, is placed within medical images such as MRI or CT scans. The technique employs LSBs of pixel values, hence the patient information is embedded without compromising the original quality of the image 1. The technique offers a natural and visually non-intrusive way of ensuring data protection since medical imaging is increasingly applied in healthcare [21]. For example, prescription information or diagnosis could be embedded within X-ray or ultrasound images. Several methods have been proposed, such as spatial domain techniques such as LSB substitution and frequency domain techniques like fast Fourier transform and discrete cosine transform (DCT), for protection against data robbery.

Text steganography often involves the hiding of secret information within text documents whereby the text to be viewed does not differ. Some of these techniques include manipulated font, changes in spacing, and format changes for embedding hidden messages within clinical documents or reports. For example, patient identifiers and medical record data are hidden in research papers or in clinical notes where the existence of such sensitive information will go undetected even if a leaking document has been intercepted. This way, sensitive information is disclosed confidentially and the integrity of the text that is visible to the user is preserved [22].

Audio steganography involves concealing messages in audio signals making it useful for encrypting voice in telemedicine and medical consultations. The most frequent techniques are LSB modification and phase coding with the help of which confidential patient data can be put into records. With steganography, there will be the privacy and confidentiality of discussions during patients' consultations, as well as the integrity of the healthcare information. This is particularly crucial as telemedicine relies more on digital audio communication [22].

Day-to-day advancement in technology has led to the development of a hybrid technology that incorporates more than one technique and encryption algorithm in steganography by embedding health information. Specifically in hybrid applications, it is possible to encrypt the medical record first before embedding the record within the images or any other data format. This double-layer protection helps to keep the embedded data safe even if it becomes known to outsiders—the data will be encoded and thus unusable until the decryption codes are provided. Besides improving the security of the data collected this approach also guarantees compliance with data protection rules in the health sector [22].

The most advanced technique is DNA-based steganography, where the data can be encoded in a sequence of DNA. With its advancement toward personalized medicine and genomics, DNA sequences can now be regarded as new mediums for hiding confidential healthcare information [23]. According to the conversion of binary data into nucleotide sequences, the patient's records can be embedded in genetic data files, which entail a very secure technique for maintaining personal medical information [24].

The process of embedding data associated with the flow of healthcare into network traffic was steganography on networks [25]. This involves concealing data in unused or possibly altered fields in the network protocol like TCP/IP headers [26]. That is, the technique can result in protected data transfer between healthcare networks. Thus, it can be used for conducting telemedicine consultations and sharing EHRs between providers [26].

Biometric Steganography Patient-specific biometric data, in the form of a fingerprint or an iris scan, is combined with health-related hidden information [26].

To embed data, this method uses images of biometrics as the medium, while the other method uses biometric patterns as keys for encrypting sensitive information [27]. Being an age where biometrics are increasingly being used for patient identification in healthcare, this method is the most secure way of keeping patient data [26].

Although steganography offers many significant benefits in protecting healthcare data, it shares similar problems that associated conventional security systems have. Because payloads are fairly large for massive data such as that found in healthcare information storage, efficiency is crucial as large payloads can alter the quality of the cover medium, a significant concern when the application has to do with imaging in the medical domain. At times, the capacity for concealing can also depend on the nature of the covering medium used [22]. Additionally, advancements in steganalysis through detection require innovations in steganographic techniques to still be effective against unauthorized data discovery [22].

In the rapidly evolving development of communication technology, AI and ML are also taking a thrilling new frontier into healthcare through integration into steganography. AI improves both the efficiency and security of data-hiding techniques. Future research will involve creating more advanced algorithms that would adaptively select their own cover media and encoding methods to maximize the confidentiality of sensitive medical information while facing the challenging realities of detection and data capacity [22].

Indeed, healthcare data is susceptible to a wide range of threats, which pose a danger to patient safety and, also the integrity and effectiveness of the delivery of healthcare. In any case, reliance on outdated systems; inadequate proper controls on access, including third-party services and IoT devices, along inappropriately compromised access controls, can all risk everything above. The breach impact is viewed to be at a severe level: in fact, breaches of patient data can cause damage in terms of reputation and financial damage to the health organization. Proactive measures are required to be taken against the countermeasures to these weaknesses and vulnerabilities to increase the cyber-resilience of the healthcare sector.

Legacy software and systems are the most vulnerable areas for the healthcare sector. Mostly, legacy systems lack security patches and support updates to defend the emerging threats, hence becoming vulnerable to exploitation by cyber adversaries [28]. Presently, the health sector is well represented by hospitals and clinics using systems unsupported by vendors, making things worse and pushing the likelihood of data breaches [28].

Poor access controls and authentication mechanisms have several weaknesses that may lead to unauthorized access and data compromise. In addition, weak password policies, sharing credentials, and poor authentication protocols compromise the integrity of access controls and provide cyber criminals with specific weaknesses that they exploit to gain access to sensitive systems [28]. The effects of compromised access controls are quite severe such that unauthorized individuals gain access to patient records and critical infrastructure and put patient confidentiality and safety at risk [28].

The use of third-party vendors brings a lot of risk factors to healthcare organizations as we have seen. Healthcare organizations include an average of 1320 vendors and are vulnerable to third-party data breaches with numerous third-party access points [29]. Many of these vendors fail to put proper security measures in place and this makes them vulnerable to cyber attackers who will access the parent company's data. It is also worth mentioning that 55% of healthcare organizations stated that they experienced a third-party data breach within the last 12 months [30].

As healthcare organizations increasingly store sensitive data in the cloud, they become more vulnerable to cloud breaches. Approximately 73% of healthcare organizations maintain sensitive data in cloud environments, and 61% have experienced attacks on their cloud infrastructure within the past year, with phishing identified as the most prevalent form of breach [3]. The lack of adequate staffing and expertise in cloud security amplifies the risk associated with cloud storage solutions [3].

In the context of the healthcare domain, the issue of data protection is urgent because a lot of such data is exchanged over the internetworking and is quite sensitive since it concerns people's medical records. Conventional cryptosystems are efficient for hiding data but fail to mask the fact that there is data to be concealed, making it prone to attracting Unwanted visitors/vulnerabilities. The opposite, steganography, applies itself to the situation where sensitive information is hidden within the seemingly unrelated text, voice, or picture. This kind of layer of security means that not even if one finds out that there is data steganographed in the cover medium cannot access it because one only gets the decryption keys right.

8.3 HEALTHCARE DATA AND ITS SECURITY CONCERNS

Healthcare data security is of paramount importance in safeguarding sensitive patient information against unauthorized access, data breaches, and evolving cyber threats. The healthcare sector faces numerous challenges, such as outdated systems, inadequate security measures for medical devices, and the increasing sophistication of cyber-attacks. Healthcare organizations need to implement robust cybersecurity strategies that encompass regulatory compliance and proactive risk management.

HIPAA security of electronic data implies that confidential medical records and other PHI must be protected from being read, written, or modified by anyone who does not have the right to do so. All these are very crucial for maintenance of the patient privacy, security of healthcare practices, and meeting the legal requirements. All these are working toward maintaining confidentiality, protecting the integrity of healthcare services as well as ensuring that the organization comes up with the regulations.

8.3.1 Types of Healthcare Data

In healthcare systems, data is rather diverse in type. In reality, it's actually of many types, which critically require patient care, administrative functions, and research. However, patient safety, particularly patient confidentiality, requires that data be protected against breaches. Adding steganography to protection should well enhance these data types' security since sensitive information can be well hidden within non-sensitive mediums.

Healthcare information can be documented in different types of forms. All the different types of healthcare forms serve important functions in patient care, medical research, and healthcare administration. All the above types of healthcare forms contribute to the basic components of designing innovative, efficient, and safe healthcare systems. The seven major kinds of healthcare information are depicted in Figure 8.2.

- *EHRs and Electronic Medical Records (EMRs)*: EHRs and EMRs have transformed how healthcare providers manage patient information. EMRs are digital versions of a patient's paper chart within one practice and include medical and treatment histories [32]. EHRs provide a more comprehensive view by sharing information with other healthcare organizations, including laboratories, specialists, medical imaging facilities, pharmacies, emergency facilities, and clinics [32].
- *Administrative Data*: Administrative data is generated during interactions with the healthcare system, including doctor visits, diagnostic procedures, hospital admissions, care facility interactions, home care, and pharmaceutical prescriptions. This data, primarily collected for administrative or billing purposes, can also be utilized to analyze healthcare delivery, cost-effectiveness, and system efficiency [32].
- *Claims Data*: Claims data consists of billable interactions between insured patients and the healthcare system. This data includes patient diagnoses, procedures, tests conducted, service dates, costs, and service locations. Leveraging claims data alongside other real-world data opens avenues for healthcare research, such as evaluating treatment effectiveness and improving medication safety [32].
- *Patient/Disease Registries*: Patient or disease registries collect data associated with patients who have specific conditions, diseases, or procedures.

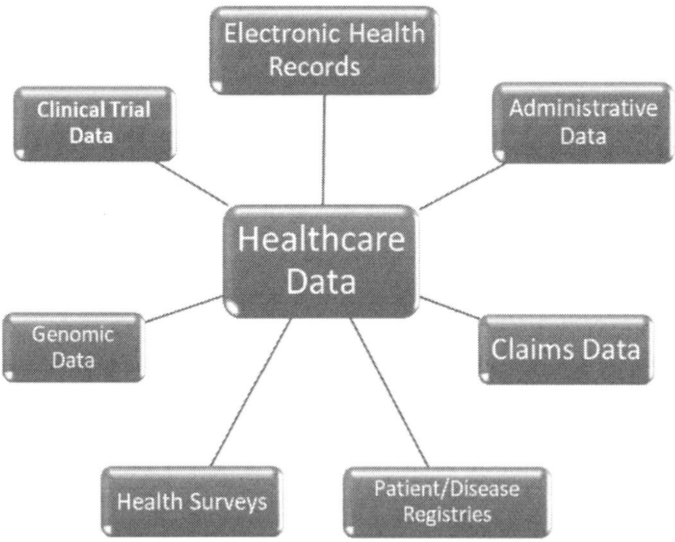

FIGURE 8.2 Types of healthcare data [31].

These registries are vital for post-marketing surveillance of pharmaceuticals and monitoring chronic conditions like Alzheimer's, cancer, diabetes, heart disease, and asthma. Registries vary in complexity, from basic spreadsheets to complex online databases accessible across organizations [32].

- *Health Surveys*: National health surveys are used to describe the health status of a population and the prevalence of diseases. They provide actual information on the epidemiological condition, trends, ways of living, and perceptions of patients about healthcare services. Some of them are the National Medical Expenditure Survey and the National Health and Nutrition Examination Survey [33].
- *Clinical Trial Data*: It comes from research studies evaluating medical, surgical, or behavioral treatments. This data is crucial for exploring disease detection methods, preventive health strategies, and improving the quality of life for patients with severe or chronic conditions. Registries like ClinicalTrials.gov provide access to databases of clinical trials [34].
- *Genomic Data*: Genomic data involves the arrangement and operation of an organism's genome, including the molecular sequence of genes, gene roles, regulatory elements, and gene interactions. This data supports genomic data science, merging genetics, computational biology, and statistical data analysis to investigate diseases and develop new treatments [32].

8.4 FRAMEWORK FOR SECURING HEALTHCARE DATA

The safeguarding of healthcare information is of prime importance because it protects not only the confidential health records of patients but also the trust that exists between the patients and their providers. The importance of keeping healthcare data secure extends to data identification and classification, data access control, data encryption, staff education, and incident management. These are discussed in greater detail in this report along concerning several current regulatory and best practices. The following is an explanation of the approach toward management and protection of healthcare data as illustrated in Figure 8.3.

- *Data Governance in Healthcare—Reliant on Very Strong Data Governance*: The healthcare industry relies strongly on robust data governance; hence the health sector must have comprehensive policies and procedures regarding how data will be collected, stored, used, and transmitted. This will be the bedrock from which the health sector is managed ethically and securely, combined with regulatory standards. Ownership and accountability are the other crucial aspects of data governance whereby the roles and responsibilities are well defined among patients, healthcare providers, and insurance entities. Data stewardship is found by assigning people or teams to lead the process of responsible and ethical management of healthcare data. Good data lifecycle management sees formulated policies guide the collection, maintenance, archiving, and eventual disposal of data. Data classification is also essential; it refers to the ranking of different types of healthcare data considering their sensitivity levels; this encompasses PII and PHI.

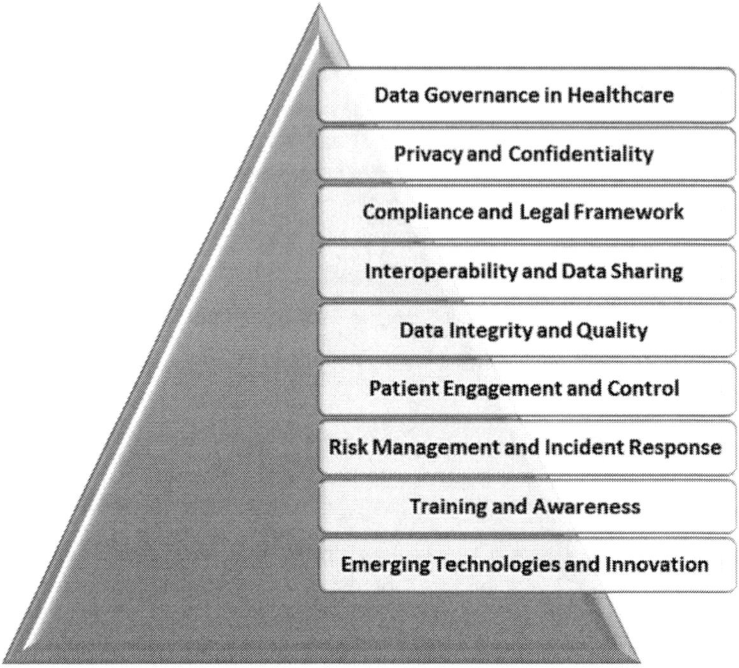

FIGURE 8.3 Framework for securing healthcare data [35].

Such practices promote a trustworthy environment enhancing patient care while protecting privacy and upholding legal demands [36].

- *Privacy and Confidentiality*: Privacy and confidentiality are very vital aspects of the patient while handling health information/data in an organization. It is privacy that concerns the right of an individual to control the access of his or her data, while confidentiality deals with only disclosing information to those authorized personnel. Key features include informed consent, whereby patients are required to permit the collection, use, and sharing of their data in full awareness of its purpose and potential risks. Data minimization practice as such ensures that one only obtains and uses data that is necessary for specified purposes. Techniques that protect patient identity by actually removing or masking PII from datasets include anonymization and pseudonymization. Strong access controls are necessary to limit access to sensitive information only to those who are formally authorized concerning the roles they play.
- *Data Security*: Healthcare management makes use of data security as a means to avoid unauthorized entry and access, data breaches, and cyberattacks. Extensive security policies along with related technologies have to begin with the data lifecycle, which covers data collection, storage, transmission, and sharing. Some of the important measures are to encrypt the data both at rest as well as during transition so that no unauthorized

access is made. Multi-factor authentication will further add to its guarantee that the individuals trying to access sensitive healthcare data are authenticated using multiple forms of verification. Role-Based Access Control will enforce permission based on user roles in healthcare organizations. IDS and firewalls will be used to monitor unauthorized access. Continuous audits and monitoring of access to data with a view to detection of any anomalies or misuse would also be carried out [21, 37].

- *Compliance and Legal Framework*: So compliance and legal issues, for instance, healthcare centers will operate in an environment that is bound by tight laws and policies that govern the management, storage, and security of healthcare information. Therefore, compliance is the aspect of engaging with the available laws and/or standards. There are a plethora of regulations and laws that are key in the operation of healthcare institutions such as the Content Insurance Portability Accountability Act which has laid down rules of conduct concerning the safeguarding of patient data on a national level especially concerning EHRs. For instance, the European Union has been more than active in putting in place some of the toughest measures against the use and abuse of personal data, including health records. HITECH also tries to broaden the existing HIPAA laws by advocating the utilization of the electronic health board and placing other requirements noticeable in cases of information compromise. Safe handling of healthcare information is not only regulated by national laws on the misuse of patient data but also includes other policies geared toward the same objectives as the CA's PHIPA [38].
- *Interoperability and Data Sharing*: Interoperability enhances the safe and effective sharing of healthcare information across systems, providers, and regions to build on better patient care, fewer errors in the medical field, and research support. Some major components will be: setting standards through systems of EHRs to standardize access to and share of patient data among healthcare providers. APIs facilitate secure data exchange among multiple systems while standards in place, such as Fast Healthcare Interoperability Resources (FHIR), advance the electronic exchange of healthcare information. Safety Exchange Protocols: Safe protocols involving HL7 and DICOM-based data exchange standards must guide the passage of healthcare data between systems [36].
- *Data Integrity and Quality*: Data integrity mirrors the accuracy and consistency of healthcare data at all stages of its life cycle. This is mainly fundamental in patient care, research, and decision-making. The main elements that guarantee data integrity revolve around validation, where data is verified periodically to ascertain whether it is complete and accurate, besides having the establishment of audit trails that monitor data transactions to track the changes or access made. Measures of data accuracy include patient record error discovery and correction. Data governance frameworks should include measures to address data quality as part of an overarching management plan to help ensure healthcare organizations remain observant about achieving high data integrity standards [36].

- *Patient Engagement and Control*: Patients must be included in controlling their health information, especially since it is the two issues that are being contested—their rights as well as their control. Patients should oversee who accesses, shares, and uses their information. Some of the enablers are patient portals, enabling e-access to one's health record, for example, lab results and prescriptions. Patients have rights on their data and are allowed to transfer them securely to any other healthcare providers. Additionally, the organizations should provide the patients with information on breaches or misuse of data and sensitize them on the handling processes involving their data [39].
- *Risk Management and Incident Response*: Effective healthcare data management must include the means for identifying risks as well as methods in case of breach or disaster, including proper planning for disaster recovery in case of prompt recovery of one's data after an incident. The regular assessment of risks determines vulnerabilities, which forms a key component in managing risks. There are additional components, such as disaster recovery, in case of prompt recovery of one's data after an incident. Incident response plans are necessary to outline procedures that one would be required to follow in case their data is breached, including the notification and secure information compromised. Another significant area of risk management is checking the compliance of third-party vendors in security and privacy standards to mitigate exposures from external exposures.
- *Training and Awareness*: An effective data management framework requires training staff and stakeholders continuously about best practices for data security and privacy policies. This includes an awareness program for security, which provides continuous training on the identification of threats, phishing, and proper handling of data. In this case, legal awareness and sensitivity training will refer to the need to ensure that employees know different laws and regulatory frameworks such as HIPAA and GDPR to name a few through giving them compliance training. Also, suggestions should be made on how employees can be trained in how to identify incidences of security threats and report them.
- *Emerging Technologies and Innovation*: Emerging technologies, including blockchain, AI, and ML, are revolutionizing the management and security of healthcare data. Key components include utilizing blockchain technology to ensure data integrity and security in transactions and establishing a tamper-proof record of data exchanges. The use of AI is also advisable for threat detection in real-time, as the AI can analyze and define whether these or those patterns are irregular and when a breach may occur. Furthermore, cloud computing provides opportunities for secure, scalable data storage and management, emphasizing adherence to stringent security protocols and compliance with regulations.

This all-around framework of management for healthcare data would make the dealing of sensitive medical information a planned affair. The focus on data governance, privacy, security, compliance, interoperability, patient engagement, and technological innovation would help healthcare organizations ensure the safety of data, deliver better services to patients, and comply with legislation in the best form. If implemented properly, such a framework ensures the proper use of healthcare data, enhances healthcare outcomes, and promotes research in the medical field.

8.4.1 Hiding Data in Images

Image steganography is perhaps the most common type of steganography applied in the pixel space of an image. That has further subdivided into sub-techniques, such as LSB modification, wherein the LSBs of the pixel values are modified to present secret messages, and much more complicated methods, for example, wavelet transforms working on the frequency domain. In healthcare, image steganography is especially useful for the concealment of sensitive patient information within medical imaging files such as MRI or CT scans. The entire process is depicted in Figure 8.4. Healthcare providers can securely send material by embedding patient IDs or diagnostic information directly into such images, thereby further protecting the personal identification of patients who receive telemedicine sessions or digital referrals.

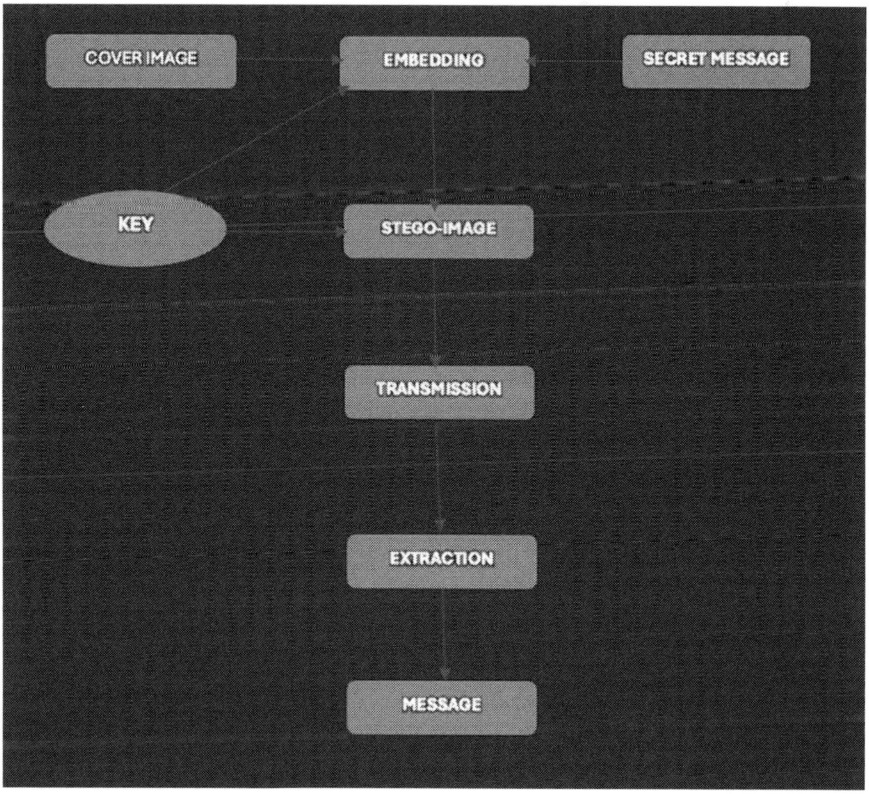

FIGURE 8.4 Hiding data in images [5].

8.4.2 Hiding Data in Text

In text steganography, secret information is encoded within text files by varying some of the attributes such as punctuations, spaces, or altering letters at regular intervals in particular positions [21, 37]. Examples of popular methods include message embedding inside the nth letter in every word or variations of font sizes and styles [40]. This approach can be very helpful in health-related situations, wherein crucial information such as a prescription or patient's background could be safely encapsulated within clinical documents. The method above, in Figure 8.5 [38] enables secure data transfer between medical practitioners in ways that do not alert the concerned data to any potential violation of its integrity while involved in e-document interactions.

8.4.3 Hiding Data in Audio

Rapid and sudden increase in the transmission of digital data over the Internet forced researchers to enhance the security system. Various alternatives are presented in this regard like cryptography, and watermarking. However, steganography has gained much importance in this context [42]. Audio steganography involves concealing data within audio files through techniques such as modifying the LSBs of audio samples or employing echo hiding, where data is embedded within echoes that are imperceptible to the listener. In healthcare, audio steganography can be used to embed patient-related audio instructions or consultative data within recordings of medical discussions or telemedicine sessions. This method shown in Figure 8.6 [43] enables the discreet transmission of sensitive information without risking exposure to unauthorized observers, thereby enhancing privacy in communications.

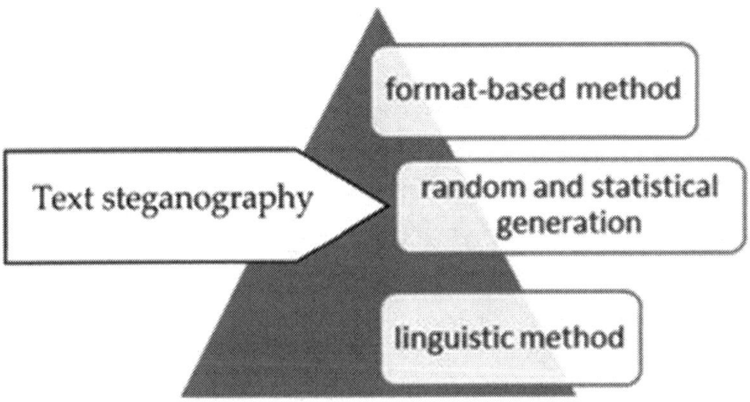

FIGURE 8.5 Hiding data in text [41].

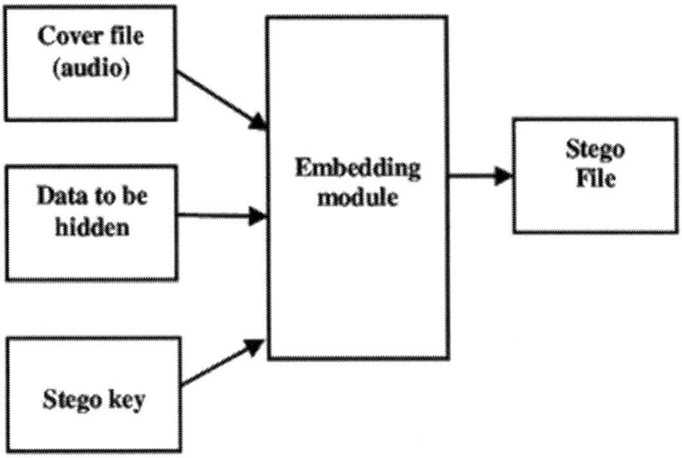

FIGURE 8.6 Hiding data in audio [43, 44].

8.4.4 Hiding Data in Video

Video steganography encompasses all the concepts related to image steganography combined with further challenges arising from the dynamic nature of video data [40]. Techniques include encoding data in specific frames or frame-based LSB or DCTs as depicted in Figure 8.7 [39]. This may also be very useful in the medical fields where there is a requirement for patient's basic information to be stored in videos recording any kind of medical treatment or educational videos. This way, sensitive information will remain confidential and only be accessed by authorized personnel, which would therefore enable one to efficiently function in passing down the information [40].

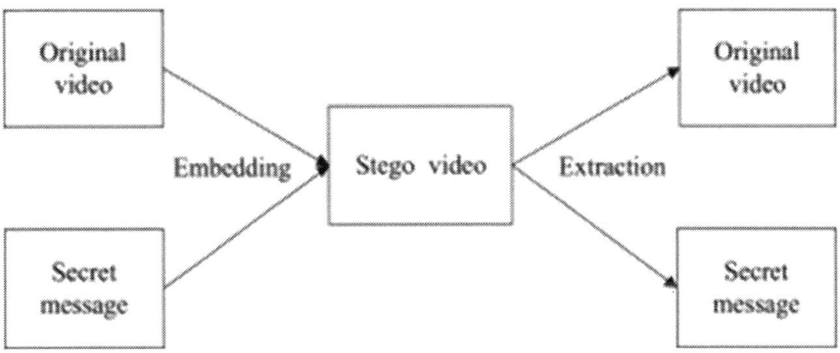

FIGURE 8.7 Hiding data in video [45].

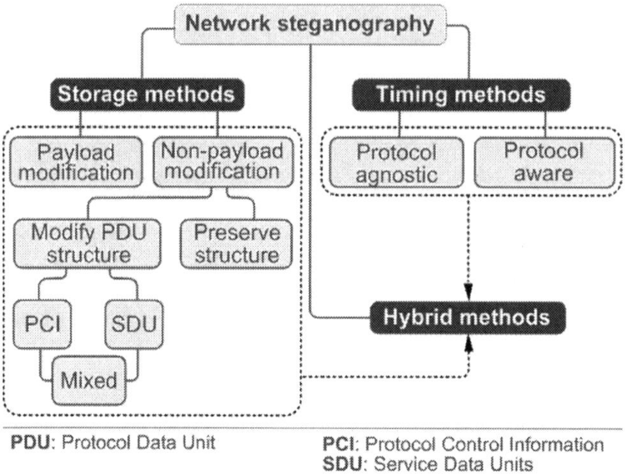

FIGURE 8.8 Hiding data in network [47].

8.4.5 Hiding Data in Network

Network steganography conceals data in network communication protocols by leveraging such things as IP addresses or packet headers to effectively utilize the messiness of network communication to obscure transmitted information [34] (Figure 8.8 [44]). This is particularly useful in healthcare in ensuring that EHRs transmitted over networks remain confidential [46]. This added layer of security is important to hospitals and clinics since they depend on a strong data system in its transmission for the protection of patient information from unauthorized access while being transferred [46].

8.4.6 Combining Steganography with Encryption

The application of steganography with encryption is one of the best approaches to raising security levels [48]. In this two-layer model, data is first encrypted, and then it is hidden in the carrier media [48]. This means that even if someone were to find the concealed information, they would not be able to understand it without the corresponding decryption key [46]. This integrated approach focuses on information security in the healthcare system due to the need to transmit protected details like patient files or essential health information [49]. With the alternate use of security measures such as the Data Encryption Standard (DES) with steganographic systems, data is not only hidden but also secured from any unlawful access during communication [25, 46].

8.5 FUTURE DIRECTIONS IN HEALTHCARE DATA

Steganography, or the art of hiding the existence of information in other, not suspicious data, begins to be implemented in the field of healthcare as an innovation in protecting data from unauthorized access and non-disclosure regarding the patient. The amount of information and its complexity are increasing day by day inside the healthcare sector EHR, genomics, and even data of wearable devices, for instance thus, the urgent need for strengthening security measures is what the sector has entered. Future directions that research is taking to pursue in steganography about healthcare data are described as under:

- *Advanced Steganography Methods*: Experts remain focused on the evolution of advanced methods in steganography techniques, often merging chaotic functions, DNA-based methods, and other new approaches to provide enhanced security with low distortion levels on the image. Advanced methods are predicted to create robust systems that ensure high-quality images with confidentially preserved embedded sensitive patient information [49, 50].
- *The Minimization of the Diagnostic Impact* area of research is to ensure that the secret information is embedded within the medical image without impairing its integrity in the diagnostic sense. IWT, among other techniques, has been studied for embedding data within the non-region-of-interest areas of the image, thereby retaining the critical quality necessary for proper medical diagnosis [5, 33, 34, 38, 39, 41, 42, 43, 44, 49, 50, 51, 52].
- *Interdisciplinary Approaches*: The fusion of steganography with other security-related technologies, such as cryptography, further strengthens data protection in the healthcare industry. The embedding of encrypted data inside medical images offers double protection and makes it highly challenging for any unauthorized parties to extract or manipulate sensitive information [4, 49].
- *AI and ML*: The usage of AI and ML would decide the best utilization of their technology in steganography for embedding and detecting the data. For instance, Support Vector Machines are used to categorize the pixels in medical images, and thus this secret information can be embedded in an extremely subtle way without any visual effects on the diagnostic value of the images [18, 52].
- *Better Interoperability with IoT Devices*: As IoT is progressively being integrated with health services, the future steganographic techniques are being designed in such a way as to ensure that this method is fully interoperable with numerous IoT devices. Such strategies will make smooth data transfer easy while further guaranteeing the safe embedding of patient details within the interface of IoT. Ultimately, in the long run, the entire issue of healthcare data security will be improved [4, 49].
- *Real-Time Steganography*: Advances in real-time steganographic systems are another of the prime concerns. The real challenge for these systems is the in-place management of embedding and extraction of data while maintaining privacy and integrity. It aims at efficient real-time transfer of data with no degradation in image quality as in healthcare applications that require modern methodologies [51].
- *Improving Data Quality and Standardization*: The proper use of steganography in healthcare is highly dependent on data quality. Future projects focus their efforts on forming standards for data harvesting that could be consistent and minimize variability, especially in unstructured data formats, to ensure reliability and effectiveness across different healthcare systems [25, 49].

- *Empowerment of Health Professionals*: There is now an acknowledgment of the need to educate and sensitize health professionals on the implications and applications of steganography in data security. Adequate training programs will be directed toward equipping these health professionals with skills and know-how that will facilitate their step-by-step implementation in health services delivery, hence ensuring confidentiality on patients' matters and better service delivery [49].

Through these guidelines, the health sector will realize a total exploitation of the potential steganography holds to ensure the safety of patient data. This further complements the objectives mentioned above in improving patient outcomes and also healthcare delivery systems.

8.6 CHALLENGES IN HEALTHCARE DATA

The steganographic approach in healthcare data is not without difficulty. An aspect of such medical image or file embedding, which entails hiding text, is the need to maintain data level. Any change would result in discrepancies regarding clinical outcomes. Apart from that, laws like HIPAA make it hard to integrate steganography in these clinical environments. Security and ease of access can hardly be achieved and correlated due to excessive encryption most likely leads to delayed retrieval of necessary information in urgent situations. On top of that, the undertaking to examine or employ steganographic tools may overburden the already overworked healthcare information technology systems. Furthermore, there is still a long way to go before the interchangeability of varying health systems is put into practice.

- *Confidentiality and Integrity*: The most important thing to preserve in the framework of the healthcare system while following steganography is ensuring that medical data, particularly the sensitive ones is private and integrity-ensured. Or, in more categorical terms, embedding the secret information efficiently without affecting the healthcare image's diagnostic quality. This is very challenging indeed for healthcare providers to ensure a proper balance between information safeguarding and accessibility as well as the accuracy of medical data.
- *Image Distortion*: Most existing steganographic methods carry considerable visible distortion in the cover images, which could deteriorate performance in clinical decision-making. The big challenge is to keep the visual fidelity required for accurate diagnostics under the embedded secret data.
- *Security against Advanced Threats*: Another challenge in implementing steganography in healthcare is the evolving sophistication of cyber threats. In addition to unnoticeable data, it would demand protection against advanced hacking methods by means of which it could be the more demanding protection, the harder the task of developing an effective steganographic system. The information would remain exposed if protective measures were not intense.

- *Traceability*: For medical applications, traceability is considered essential for audits and compliance. Design of a steganographic process wherein data is being embedded in a way that the presence of data to be tracked should not leave any hints at all is a very complex task and one of the challenging tasks to achieve such functionality and remain confidential too. Accountability has to be built through determinable methods.
- *Capacity versus Security*: It is a challenge to bring the right balance between the data-hiding capacity of steganographic methods and information security. Systems providing enough storage and concealment abilities lack security provisions, and those that prioritize security may not support large volumes well.
- *Data Management and Standardization*: Effective management of these diverse data sets of healthcare, which include images and EHRs, is still very problematic. This type of heterogeneous data is in need of advanced management systems integrated with standardization protocols to perfect the process and heighten interoperability among several systems.

8.7 CONCLUSION

This chapter focuses attention on the great need for intensified data protection in the digitized health services of the country, as increasingly sensitive information about patients is now exposed to emerging cyber threats. Though traditional encryption is a necessity, it cannot provide adequate resistive power to more complex attacks. Steganography is a critical addition to the security process because it conceals any sensitive information in an innocuous-looking medium like images and audio, or text, whose functionality does not suggest the presence of hidden information. The most promising techniques are related to advanced methods, such as LSB embedding, DNA-based methods, and neural network-driven steganography. These will benefit the preservation of the diagnostic utility of medical images and biological signals, such as ECGs. Notwithstanding all these efforts, there is a challenge: image distortion, computational overhead, and compliance with healthcare regulations, such as HIPAA and GDPR need to be addressed. If ML was utilized with these more advanced algorithms, it may result in better efficiency and resilience against detection. Future work would focus on optimizing these approaches and eventually implementing them in a way that makes steganography as non-intrusive as possible to the healthcare systems, hopefully minimizing breach risks for patient confidentiality and enhancing trust in digital health environments.

REFERENCES

1. Murray, J. (2024). *The Importance of Data Security in Healthcare.* Enterprise Guardian® | EnGuard®. https://www.enguard.com/data-security-in-healthcare/
2. Islam, T. (2024). *5 Consequences of Data Breach in Healthcare.* ComplyAssistant. https://www.complyassistant.com/resources/tips/the-ripple-effects-of-data-breaches-in-healthcare-a-closer-look/
3. GeeksforGeeks. (2023). *Image Steganography in Cryptography - GeeksforGeeks.* GeeksforGeeks. https://www.geeksforgeeks.org/image-steganography-in-cryptography/

4. Hashim, M. M., Rhaif, S. H., Abdulrazzaq, A. A., Ali, A. H., & Taha, M. S. (2020). Based on IoT healthcare application for medical data authentication: Towards a new secure framework using steganography. IOP Conference Series Materials Science and Engineering, 881(1), 012120. https://doi.org/10.1088/1757-899x/881/1/012120
5. Majeed, M. A., Sulaiman, R., Shukur, Z., & Hasan, M. K. (2021). A review on text steganography techniques. Mathematics, 9(21), 2829. https://doi.org/10.3390/math9212829
6. 3 July 2024. (2024). *The Importance of Data Privacy in Healthcare*. tigahealth.com. https://www.tigahealth.com/the-importance-of-data-privacy-in-healthcare/
7. Kariotis, T. C., Prictor, M., Chang, S., & Gray, K. (2022). Impact of electronic health records on information practices in mental health contexts: Scoping review. Journal of Medical Internet Research. https://doi.org/10.2196/30405
8. Data Breaches: In the Healthcare Sector. (2021). CIS. https://www.cisecurity.org/blog/data-breaches-in-the-healthcare-sector/
9. Semilof, M. (2023). *What is steganography?* | Definition from TechTarget. TechTarget. https://www.techtarget.com/searchsecurity/definition/steganography
10. Contributors to Wikimedia projects. (2024). *Steganography - Wikipedia*. Wikimedia Foundation, Inc. https://en.wikipedia.org/wiki/Steganography
11. Li, L., Zhou, J., Gao, Z., Hua, W., Fan, L., Yu, H., Hagen, L., Zhang, Y., Assimes, T.L., Hemphill, L., & Ma, S. (2024). A scoping review of using Large Language Models (LLMs) to investigate Electronic Health Records (EHRs). ArXiv, abs/2405.03066.
12. Tiga Health. (n.d.). *The Importance of Data Privacy in Healthcare*. Retrieved September 12, 2024, from https://www.tigahealth.com/the-importance-of-data-privacy-in-healthcare/
13. Sreeja, C.S. (2013). A Model for the Secured Data Transfer of Healthcare Data by Image Steganography and Cryptography Techniques. https://www.semanticscholar.org/paper/d6de70b9ea1648fd369037b6bcb4fc540d74531c
14. Haverkamp, I., & Sarmah, D. K. (2024). "Evaluating the merits and constraints of cryptography-steganography fusion: A systematic analysis." International Journal of Information Security, May 5, 2024. https://doi.org/10.1007/s10207-024-00853-9
15. Hua, C., et al. (2023). "Steganography for medical record image." Computers in Biology and Medicine. https://doi.org/10.1016/j.compbiomed.2023.107344.
16. Haverkamp, I., & Sarmah, D. K. (2024). Evaluating the merits and constraints of cryptography-steganography fusion: A systematic analysis. International Journal of Information Security. https://doi.org/10.1007/s10207-024-00853-9
17. Rajendran, S., Kulkarni, V., Chaudhari, S., & Gupta, P. K. (2020). An update on medical data steganography and encryption. Advances in Intelligent Systems and Computing. https://doi.org/10.1007/978-981-15-2740-1_13
18. Chowdhuri, P., Pal, P., & Si, T. (2023). A novel steganographic technique for medical image using SVM and IWT. Multimedia Tools and Applications, 82(13), 20497–20516. https://doi.org/10.1007/s11042-022-14301-0
19. Anandha, R. D. A., de La Croix, N. J., & Ahmad, T. (2023). "A Steganographic Scheme to Protect Medical Data Using Radiological Images," 2023 IEEE 15th International Conference on Computational Intelligence and Communication Networks (CICN), Bangkok, Thailand, pp. 369–374, ieee.org, September 12, 2024. https://ieeexplore.ieee.org/document/10402248
20. Subramanian, N., Elharrouss, O., Al-Maadeed, S., & Bouridane, A. (2021). "Image steganography: A review of the recent advances. IEEE Access, 9, 23409–23423. https://ieeexplore.ieee.org/document/9335027
21. Vazquez, E., Torres, S., Sanchez, G., Avalos, J.-G., Abarca, M., Frias, T., Juarez, E., Trejo, C., & Hernandez, D. (2022). Confidentiality in medical images through a genetic-based steganography algorithm in artificial intelligence. Frontiers in Robotics and AI. https://doi.org/10.3389/frobt.2022.1031299

22. Ogundokun, R. O., & Abikoye, O. C. (2021). A safe and secured medical textual information using an improved LSB image steganography. International Journal of Digital Multimedia Broadcasting. https://doi.org/10.1155/2021/8827055
23. Al-Ahmadi, W. E., Aljahdali, A. O., Thabit, F., & Munshi, A. (2024). A secure fingerprint hiding technique based on DNA sequence and mathematical function. *PeerJ Computer Science*. https://doi.org/10.7717/peerj-cs.1847
24. Esmaeelzadeh Rostam, H., Motameni, H., & Enayatifar, R. (2023). Privacy-preserving in the smart healthcare system using steganography and chaotic functions based on DNA. Security and Privacy. https://doi.org/10.1002/spy2.363
25. Mansour, R. F., & Girgis, M. R. (2021). Steganography-based transmission of medical images over unsecure network for telemedicine applications. Computers, Materials & Continua. https://doi.org/10.32604/cmc.2021.017064
26. McAteer, I., Ibrahim, A., Zheng, G., Yang, W., & Valli, C. (2019). Integration of biometrics and steganography: A comprehensive review. Technologies. https://doi.org/10.3390/technologies7020034
27. Jabbar, M. S., & Issa, S. S. (2023). A crypto-steganography healthcare management: Towards a secure communication channel for data COVID-19 updating. Indonesian Journal of Electrical Engineering and Computer Science. https://ijeecs.iaescore.com/index.php/IJEECS/article/download/29231/17060
28. Cogent | *Blog | Healthcare Cybersecurity: Addressing Vulnerabilities in The Medical Industry*. (2024). cogentinfo.com. https://www.cogentinfo.com/resources/healthcare-cybersecurity-addressing-vulnerabilities-in-the-medical-industry
29. Herzberg, Ben. (2023). *3 Healthcare Data Vulnerabilities to be Mindful of in 2023*. Security Magazine. https://www.securitymagazine.com/blogs/14-security-blog/post/98803-3-healthcare-data-vulnerabilities-to-be-mindful-of-in-2023
30. Kumar, V., Sharma, S., Kumar, C., & Sahu, A. K. (2023). Latest trends in deep learning techniques for image steganography. International Journal of Digital Crime and Forensics. https://doi.org/10.4018/ijdcf.318666
31. Batko, K., & Ślęzak, A. (2022). The use of big data analytics in healthcare. Journal of Big Data, 9(1). https://doi.org/10.1186/s40537-021-00553-4
32. KMS Staff. (2024). *Types of Healthcare Data: A Complete Overview*. KMS Healthcare. https://kms-healthcare.com/blog/types-of-healthcare-data/
33. Chen, J., Wu, Y., Sun, Y., & Yang, C. (2022). Image encryption algorithm using 2-order bit compass coding and chaotic mapping. Symmetry, 14(7), 1482. https://doi.org/10.3390/sym14071482
34. Seh, A.H., Zarour, M., Alenezi, M., Sarkar, A.K., Agrawal, A., Kumar, R., & Ahmad Khan, R. (2020). Healthcare data breaches: Insights and implications. Healthcare, 8, 133. https://doi.org/10.3390/healthcare8020133
35. Batko, K., & Ślęzak, A. (2022). The use of big data analytics in healthcare. Journal of Big Data, 9(1), 3. doi: 10.1186/s40537-021-00553-4. Epub 2022 Jan 6. PMID: 35013701; PMCID: PMC8733917. https://pmc.ncbi.nlm.nih.gov/articles/PMC8733917/
36. Team Atlan. (2024). *Data Governance in Healthcare: Complete Guide for 2024*. Atlan. https://atlan.com/data-governance-in-healthcare/
37. Han, S. (2023). *The Importance of Healthcare Data Security*. cprime.com. https://www.cprime.com/resources/blog/the-importance-of-healthcare-data-security/
38. Yaghobi, S. R., & Sajedi, H. (2021b). Text steganography in webometrics. International Journal of Information Technology, 13(2), 621–635. https://doi.org/10.1007/s41870-020-00572-z
39. Brown, T. (2019, April 15). Statistics on healthcare data breaches. ComplianceHome. https://www.compliancehome.com/statistics-on-healthcare-data-breaches/
40. Jamuna, A. (2022). Video steganography in the field of e-healthcare. International Journal of Research in Engineering, Science and Management, 5(7), 9–12. ISSN (Online): 2581-5792, https://www.ijresm.com

41. Text Steganography. (2014, February 1). IEEE Conference Publication | IEEE Xplore. https://ieeexplore.ieee.org/document/6798347/citations?tabFilter=papers#citations
42. Audio Steganography. (2014). In 2014 International Conference on Reliability, Optimization and Information Technology - ICROIT 2014. ("Audio Steganography," 2014, p. 2) https://doi.org/10.1109/ICROIT.2014.6798347
43. Figure 1. Basic audio Steganography. (n.d.). ResearchGate. https://www.researchgate.net/figure/Basic-audio-Steganography_fig1_282822420
44. Fig. 1 shows basic classification of network steganography methods, … (n.d.). Research Gate. https://www.researchgate.net/figure/shows-basic-classification-of-network-steganography-methods-including-new-technique_fig1_338365775
45. Kunhoth, J., Subramanian, N., & Al-Maadeed, S. et al. (2023). Video steganography: Recent advances and challenges. Multimedia Tools and Applications 82, 41943–41985. https://doi.org/10.1007/s11042-023-14844-w
46. sheki018. (2024). *GitHub - sheki018/Secure-Transmission-of-Medical-Images-using-Encryption-and-Steganography: The major contribution of this project is combining several steganography and encryption techniques, for secure transmission of data without leakage and unauthorized access.* GitHub. https://github.com/sheki018/Secure-Transmission-of-Medical-Images-using-Encryption-and-Steganography
47. Seo, J. O., Manoharan, S., & Mahanti, A., "Network steganography and steganalysis - a concise review," 2016 2nd International Conference on Applied and Theoretical Computing and Communication Technology (iCATccT), Bangalore, India, 2016, pp. 368–371, doi: 10.1109/ICATCCT.2016.7912025. keywords: {Codecs;Protocols;Games;Timing;Media;Real-time systems;Transcoding}, https://ieeexplore.ieee.org/document/7912025
48. Abdul, W. (2022). Security of medical images over insecure communication channels using zero-steganography. International Journal of Distributed Sensor Networks. https://doi.org/10.1177/15501477211006347
49. AlEisa, H. N. (2022). Data confidentiality in healthcare monitoring systems based on image steganography to improve the exchange of patient information using the internet of things. Journal of Healthcare Engineering. https://doi.org/10.1155/2022/7528583
50. Usman, M. A., & Usman, M. R., "Using image steganography for providing enhanced medical data security," 2018 15th IEEE Annual Consumer Communications & Networking Conference (CCNC), Las Vegas, NV, USA, 2018, pp. 1–4, doi: 10.1109/CCNC.2018.8319263
51. Patange, A., Mahesan, K. V., Manjula, C., Donald, C., Babu, S., Peroumal, V., & Arumugam, M. (2023). Advancements in optical steganography for secure medical data transmission in telehealth systems. Optical and Quantum Electronics. https://doi.org/10.1007/s11082-023-05080-5
52. Ahmad Bamanga, M., Kamalu Babando, A., & Ahmed Shehu, M. (2024). Recent advances in steganography. Steganography - The Art of Hiding Information [Working Title]. https://doi.org/10.5772/intechopen.1004521

9 Depression Detection Using Machine Learning Algorithms for Smart Healthcare System

Sanjay Singh, Manoj Kumar, and Urmila Pilania

9.1 INTRODUCTION

As per World Health Organization (WHO) [1], depression is a very common mental disease, disturbing around 280 million persons worldwide. Characterized by persistent sadness, loss of interest, and a range of physical and emotional symptoms, depression significantly impacts a person's quality of life, productivity, and social relationships. If treatment for depression is not taken on time then it can have serious consequences, including an increased risk of suicide [2]. Despite its global importance, many cases of depression are undiagnosed or misdiagnosed, leading to delayed intervention and inappropriate care. Early detection of depression is essential for effective treatment. However, classical diagnostic techniques are often time-consuming and rely on subjective assessments by clinical staff. Recent developments in Artificial Intelligence (AI) and natural language processing (NLP), which is utilized to computationally analyze human language [3], have opened new avenues in mental health research, particularly in the areas of automated detection and diagnosis. One promising area of research is the use of language analysis to identify patterns associated with mental illness [4].

Language reflects not only mental processes but also emotional states, making it a rich source of data for assessing psychological well-being. In the work, the author's objective is to explore the potential of utilizing multimodal data, specifically audio signals and text transcripts, for effective depression prediction using Machine Learning (ML) techniques. The author's objective is to examine whether combining speech-based audio features, such as Mel-Frequency Cepstral Coefficients (MFCC) [5], with spoken language-derived textual features can improve the ability of ML models to identify depression. Furthermore, we aim to study the performance of different ML classification techniques, such as Support Vector Machines (SVM), and Random Forest (RF) along with boosting algorithms including Gradient Boosting (GB) and Extreme Gradient Boost (XGBoost) in detecting depression patterns, thus reconnoitering the potential of a multimodal approach to enhance the accuracy and robustness of systems for mental health diagnosis assessment.

DOI: 10.1201/9781003510932-9

SVM is a popular algorithm in supervised ML that is frequently utilized for both classification purposes. The objective of SVM is to identify the best hyperplane that distinguishes information points from different classes within a space of many dimensions. RF is a general ensemble ML method that is mainly employed for tasks involving classification and regression. During training, it constructs numerous decision trees and combines their results to enhance accuracy and avoid overfitting. Boosting is a method in ML that includes merging weak learners, such as decision trees, sequentially to produce a powerful learner. Every newcomer concentrates on fixing the mistakes made by those who came before them. GB is an algorithm for boosting that reduces the loss function of the model by iterating. XGBoost improves upon GB by incorporating various optimizations and extra features to enhance performance.

9.2 RELATED WORK

Yang et al.'s RLKT-MDD framework [6] is an innovative approach to improve depression diagnosis by leveraging multimodal datasets, particularly the DAIC-WoZ (Distress Analysis Interview Corpus – Wizard-of-Oz) database. The study uniquely integrated three data modalities – 4,444 visual, audio, and textual inputs – which help in understanding the intricate nature of depression. The researchers used the Facial Action Coding System (FACS) to extract facial features which gives intuition into the emotional state of participants based on their facial expressions.

For audio features, they used COVAREP [7], a robust speech feature analysis tool that can capture various prosodic elements such as pitch and tone. Text features were processed using a BERT-style language model that effectively understands context and semantics for NLP tasks. The methodology of this study involved the initial encoding and decoding of unimodal features, which has been mixed utilizing a multi-head attention mechanism. The step was critical as it allowed the technique to focus on distinct parts of the input data, improving the representation of multimodal features. The final stage of their approach involved knowledge transfer using a pre-trained model and sentiment dataset to enhance the diagnostic capabilities of the technique. The results were promising. The framework achieved the following metrics: Accuracy – 80.20%, Recall – 81.00%, F1 score – 80.60%, and Precision – 81.10%. These outcomes highlight the potential of the proposed model for accurate diagnosis of depression and demonstrate the key advantages of integrating different modalities and using advanced ML techniques.

This study [8] introduces a new Machine Speech Chain Model for identifying Depression (MSCDR) which can extract speech features relevant to depression in a text-independent manner, enhancing recognition accuracy. The suggested MSCDR uses Learning Predictive Coding (LPC) and MFCC features to explain speech production and perception processes. Next, an alternating integration of a 1-dimensional Convolutional Neural Network (CNN) and a Long Short-Term Memory (LSTM) network is utilized for capturing both intra- and inter-segment dynamic depressive features to classify them effectively. The model is evaluated on two diverse datasets, the DAIC-Woz and the Multimodal Open Dataset for Mental Disorder Analysis, which have varying languages and paradigms. The MSCDR achieved an accuracy of 0.77 and 0.86 on the two datasets, with average F1 scores of 0.75 and 0.86, outperforming other established methods. This enhancement highlights how speech production and perception features work together to convey information about depression. The sample size has been selected very small, which could limit its use in clinical translation to a certain extent.

Ravi et al. [9] introduce four different disentanglement techniques for separating speaker-identity details from depression-related details, preventing the jeopardy of patient confidentiality – maximizing adversarial Speaker Identification (SID) loss (ADV), equalizing SID Loss with Variance (LEV), equalizing SID loss with Cross-Entropy (LECE), and equalizing SID loss with KL divergence (LEKLD). The tests, which included a variety of input features and model designs, resulted in enhanced F1 scores for detecting Major Depressive Disorder (MDD) and voice privacy qualities, as measured by Gain in Voice Distinctiveness (VD) and De-Identification Scores (DeID). Using ComparE16 features on the DAIC-WOZ dataset in English achieves the maximum F1 score of 80%, marking the top F1-Score for audio-only SOTA depression detection. Using the raw audio signal on the EATD dataset (Mandarin), ADV achieves an F1-Score of 72.38%, outperforming the current State-Of-the-Art (SOTA) multimodal approach. This approach shows a potential path for detecting depression through speech while protecting patient privacy by decreasing reliance on speaker-identity features.

Wanderley Espinola et al. [10] aims to examine the utilization of voice features as objective markers for identifying MDD and provide a more reliable alternative to traditional subjective diagnostic methods. Researchers utilized ML to identify subtle indicators of MDD by analyzing voice patterns that may indicate depression (e.g., flat tone, slow speech rate, monotony). The study included 33 participants, 22 patients have been diagnosed with MDD and 11 have been healthy controls. A random tree model was applied to detect these voice features, achieving an accuracy of 87.56% in distinguishing MDD patients from healthy participants. Supportive indices such as a kappa index of 0.75, sensitivity of 0.91, and specificity of 0.83 confirmed the reliability of the model and its agreement with clinical diagnosis. These outcomes suggest that ML in speech analysis may provide a more objective and accurate tool for detecting MDD in clinical settings.

The research [11] focuses on automatically detecting depression in Korean speakers based on acoustic features, providing a more objective approach than traditional self-diagnosis. A total of 318 participants (153 diagnosed with MDD and 165 healthy controls) were recorded reading specific passages. Because the speech patterns of depressed patients are often monotonous or slow, the researchers analyzed prosodic features like pitch, rhythm, and intonation. Three models were evaluated: classical ML techniques based on these acoustic features, a pre-trained network, and a CNN that analyzes log-mel spectrograms of deeper speech patterns. The CNN model, designed to capture complex speech features, attained a good accuracy of 78.14%. This proposes that deep learning methods may provide a more accurate tool for predicting depression, especially for non-English speakers.

Jain et al. [12] propose a hybrid AI-based method for analyzing depression that provides a more comprehensive assessment than single-modal approaches by integrating video, audio, and text features. Their model first assesses the severity of depression using the Patient Health Questionnaire (PHQ-8) with a Deep Residual Network (D-ResNet) that captures video and audio features. To deepen the analysis, a paragraph vector-based kernel extreme learning machine (PV-KELM) identifies psychometric indicators associated with depression. These PHQ-8 scores and psychometric features are processed by an ensemble classifier that combines SVM, NB, and DT methods to predict the existence of depression. Implemented in Python and tested on the DAIC-WOZ dataset, the model obtained good accuracy, precision, recall, and F-measure, as well as good RMSE, MAE, JSD, and contextual similarity metrics. The results highlight the validity of the method and its advantages compared to traditional methods for classifying depression in multimodal contexts.

9.3 PROPOSED METHODOLOGY

The librosa library is used to extract audio features like MFCC along with other important features, while transcripts of participants' speech provide the text data. Combining audio and text information produces a structured dataset that links participant IDs in both forms. The dataset contains interviews of 219 participants in the form of audio and text features. The data recording tool used in the work is an automated script that was established to effectively collect target files from a specific website to ensure a systematic and complete data call.

After the collection of data, the integration of audio with text is done for further analysis. The details of participants are fetched from the original Excel file and after fetching details data is labeled with the required fields. This is done to match the audio file with the text files. Mainly the participant's unique ID plays an important role. The audio features are retrieved from the prepared dataset by applying the bookish library, it computes MFCC along with selected features like spectral contrast and zero-crossing frequency. These selected features play an important role in capturing deviations in speech patterns that might specify emotional distress. These computed MFCCs are aggregated and kept in the form of data frames so that these frames can be utilized for analysis when required.

The text data is also filtered and stored in a single place after retrieving from CSV files. These simplified text transcripts match the recording of the particular person in audio. This multimodal dataset helps ML algorithms to achieve good results. So finally depression is predicted in the combination of audio and text data. The ML algorithms take general steps such as preprocessing, selection of features, retrieval of features, and classification. As implementation is done in Python so mainly required libraries are imported.

The authors utilized the Librosa library for the audio data. For checking depression, the emotional status of the person has been extracted. Emotional features include the MFCC coefficients, the contrast of spectrals, and the crossing rate which should be zero. These features capture the required parameters like height, tone, and rhythm. These features are combined with text which is derived from transcription. This integration of speech and text provides the most suitable way of predicting depression. Figure 9.1 represents the complete flow of the proposed work. Input is the integration of speech and text files as shown in the figure. This input is converted into vector form and then these vectors are matched in the dataset. ML models are trained on this dataset for the detection of depression.

Accuracy could be defined as the ratio of accurate predictions to the overall number of observations [13], Precision calculates the ratio of accurate positive predictions to all predicted positive instances [14], Recall is the ratio of correctly predicted positive

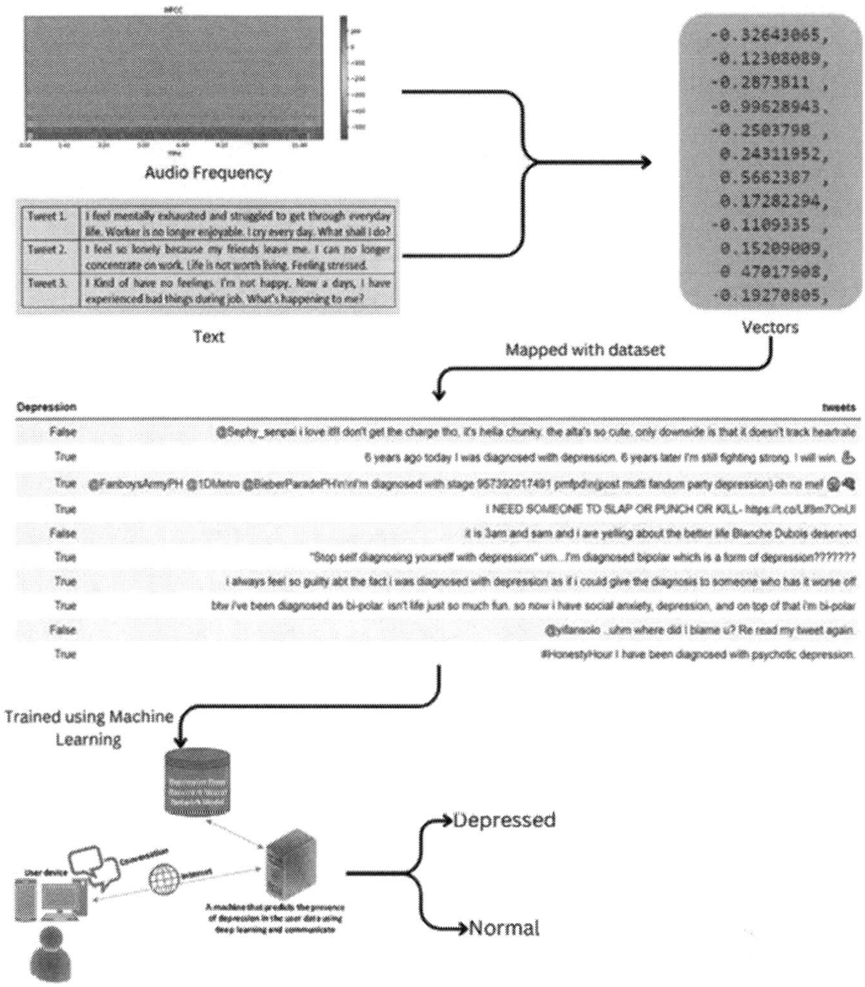

FIGURE 9.1 Model flowchart.

observations to all true positive observations [15], and The F1 Score is calculated as the harmonic average of precision and recall. It offers a combination of precision and recall, particularly in cases of imbalanced class distribution. This multimodal, data-driven methodology enables more nuanced depression detection, leveraging the complementary strengths of audio and text analytics to improve prediction accuracy.

9.4 RESULT AND DISCUSSION

The result of this method demonstrated a significant enhancement in detecting depression through the combined use of audio and text features. By employing a multimodal approach, the classification models – SVM, RF, GB, and XGBoost achieved enhanced performance compared to using a single modality alone. The dataset is

TABLE 9.1
Performance Metrics

Model	Accuracy	Precision	Recall	F1-Score
Random forest	0.71	0.73	0.96	0.76
SVM	0.73	0.74	0.96	0.78
Gradient boosting	0.73	0.75	0.93	0.76
XGBoost	0.78	0.78	0.96	0.79

built by combining MFCC, spectral contrast, and speech transcripts. This complex dataset allows the models to find better depressive states. The work is assessed by determining accuracy, precision, recall, and F1-score.

The simulation results proved that multimodal techniques outperformed traditional techniques which work only on text files as shown in Table 9.1. Although all four proposed models performed well in terms of simulation results XGBoost achieved the highest values of performance metrics.

XGBoost is good in binary classification tasks; it overtakes classical techniques by handling constraints. It uses L1 and L2 regularization for handling overfitting and provides multiprocessing for fast training. It handles the missing data without applying the preprocessing step. It works well with complex datasets by applying distributed computing. It also minimizes the use of memory. It carries functions like primary stopping, combined cross-validation, and loss function which improve model performance.

Overall, the results confirmed that combining audio and text data significantly improves the proposed work detection depression capacity, providing a more holistic analysis of the participant's emotional state. This multimodal approach as in Figure 9.2 is particularly effective because it captures both verbal content (what is said)

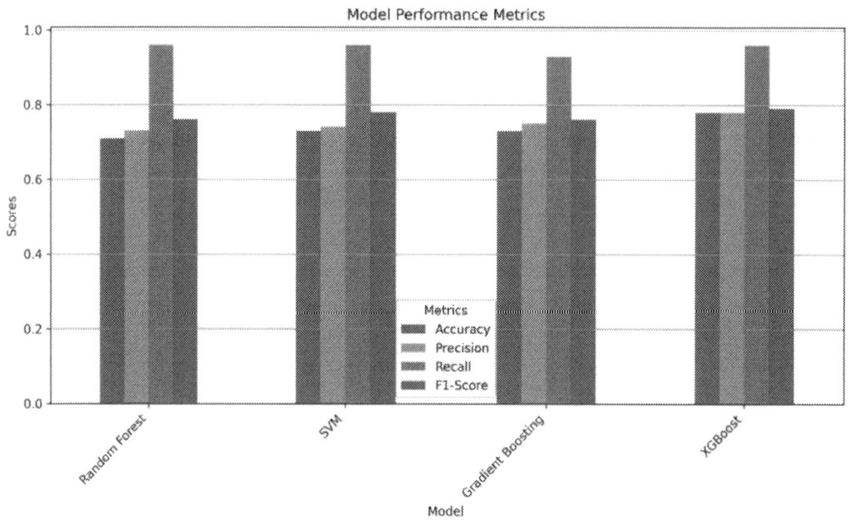

FIGURE 9.2 Comparison graph.

and paralinguistic features (how it is said), which together provide a deeper understanding of underlying psychological conditions such as depression. Among the proposed algorithms XGBoost performed best in terms of performance metrics including accuracy 78%, precision 78%, recall 96%, and F1-score 79%. It has been concluded from the proposed work that ML techniques save time, save effort, and provide more accurate results compared to traditional techniques.

9.5 CONCLUSION

The conclusion of the work underlines the effectiveness of a multimodal approach to detect depression by integrating both audio and textual data. The combination of MFCC and other audio characteristics with analysis of the vocal transcription provides a more robust and complete picture to recognize the depressive states. By exploiting both the verbal content and the characteristics of the audio signal, the automatic learning models have been able to capture subtler indicative signs of depression, obtaining greater accuracy, precision, recall, and F1 scores than the approaches to single mode. This research highlights the critical importance of multimodal data in understanding complex psychological conditions such as depression. The use of advanced classification algorithms such as SVM, RF, XGBoost, and GB further demonstrate that automatic learning techniques can be successfully applied to detect mental health conditions, opening the way to innovative diagnostic tools. XGBoost outperformed the 3 ML methods by achieving accuracy at 78%, precision at 78%, recall at 96%, and F1-score at 79%. The simulation of work highlights the potential of these methods for use in real-world applications, such as automated mental health assessments or remote monitoring systems, providing a more objective and scalable solution for early detection of depression.

REFERENCES

1. https://www.who.int/news-room/fact-sheets/detail/depression
2. https://my.clevelandclinic.org/health/diseases/9290-depression
3. Khurana, D., Koli, A., Khatter, K., & Singh, S. (2023). Natural language processing: State of the art, current trends and challenges. *Multimedia Tools and Applications*, *82*(3), 3713–3744.
4. Url: https://en.wikipedia.org/wiki/Artificial_intelligence_in_mental_health
5. Islam, M. R., Kabir, M. A., Ahmed, A., Kamal, A. R. M., Wang, H., & Ulhaq, A. (2018). Depression detection from social network data using machine learning techniques. *Health Information Science and Systems*, *6*, 1–12.
6. Yang, S., Cui, L., Wang, L., Wang, T., & You, J. (2024). Enhancing multimodal depression diagnosis through representation learning and knowledge transfer. *Heliyon*, *10*(4).
7. Degottex, G., Kane, J., Drugman, T., Raitio, T., & Scherer, S. (2014, May). COVAREP—A collaborative voice analysis repository for speech technologies. In *2014 IEEE international conference on acoustics, speech and signal processing (ICASSP)* (pp. 960–964). IEEE.
8. Du, M., Liu, S., Wang, T., Zhang, W., Ke, Y., Chen, L., & Ming, D. (2023). Depression recognition using a proposed speech chain model fusing speech production and perception features. *Journal of Affective Disorders*, *323*, 299–308.

9. Ravi, V., Wang, J., Flint, J., & Alwan, A. (2024). Enhancing accuracy and privacy in speech-based depression detection through speaker disentanglement. *Computer Speech & Language*, *86*, 101605.
10. Wanderley Espinola, C., Gomes, J. C., Mônica Silva Pereira, J., & dos Santos, W. P. (2022). Detection of major depressive disorder, bipolar disorder, schizophrenia and generalized anxiety disorder using vocal acoustic analysis and machine learning: An exploratory study. *Research on Biomedical Engineering*, *38*(3), 813–829.
11. Kim, A. Y., Jang, E. H., Lee, S. H., Choi, K. Y., Park, J. G., & Shin, H. C. (2023). Automatic depression detection using smartphone-based text-dependent speech signals: Deep convolutional neural network approach. *Journal of Medical Internet Research*, *25*, e34474.
12. Jain, S., Jacob, I. J., & Mandava, A. K. (2023). D-ResNet-PVKELM: Deep neural network and paragraph vector based kernel extreme machine learning model for multimodal depression analysis. *Multimedia Tools and Applications*, *82*(17), 25973–26004.
13. Pandey, S. K., Shekhawat, H. S., Prasanna, S. R. M., Bhasin, S., & Jasuja, R. (2022). A deep tensor-based approach for automatic depression recognition from speech utterances. *PLoS One*, *17*(8), e0272659.
14. Mazumdar, S., Dey, S., Patra, S., Mondal, S., Adhikary, A., & Paria, A. (2024, February). A Systematic Review on the Depression and Suicidal Thought Detection Using Machine Learning Based Classifiers. In *International Conference on Emerging Trends in Mathematical Sciences & Computing* (pp. 24–40). Cham: Springer Nature Switzerland.
15. Gratch, J., Artstein, R., Lucas, G. M., Stratou, G., Scherer, S., Nazarian, A., ... & Morency, L. P. (2014, May). The distress analysis interview corpus of human and computer interviews. In *LREC* (pp. 3123–3128).

10 Exploring Artificial Intelligence Techniques for Disease Outcome Prediction

Case Study and Smart Healthcare Integration

Shikha Sharma, Ajay Khunteta, Satya Prakash Awasthi, Sumit Kumar Kapoor, and Vijay Prakash Sharma

10.1 INTRODUCTION

Medicine has become the recent frontier of an unprecedented revolution in predictive modeling for disease outcomes and is part of a more significant change in the current healthcare landscape. Whether acute or chronic, diseases still challenge healthcare systems worldwide [1, 2]. Predicting disease outcomes can achieve high value in terms of patient care [3], optimized resource allocation, and improved decision-making in medical practices [4]. In this regard, data-driven insights through Artificial Intelligence (AI) make indispensable tools for improving healthcare outcomes [5, 6].

This holistic study explores the uncharted territory of predictive modeling in healthcare by AI. We understand that diseases come in variations based on genetics, lifestyle, and environmental factors, which are complex. AI's adaptive and learning capabilities significantly weigh in models specific to the disease for unprecedented accuracy [7, 8].

To understand AI's impact on predictive modeling, we provide an overview of AI techniques used in healthcare. From traditional machine learning to advanced deep neural networks, AI equips predictive models with the most diverse data sources, such as clinical records, patient profiles, medical imaging, and omics data [9–11].

Furthermore, the practical applicability of AI-based predictions also depends on their interpretability and implementation into clinical practice. We outline methods that enhance explainability in AI models, hence building trust between AI and healthcare clinicians [12–14].

DOI: 10.1201/9781003510932-10

It takes us from the current landscape into tomorrow's vision, especially toward predictive modeling in personalized medicine for early disease detection and treatment optimization. This perspective combines multimodal data fusion, federated learning, and real-time monitoring to transform healthcare into an active and patient-centric domain.

Despite these advancements, several challenges must be addressed to fully realize the potential of AI in predictive modeling for healthcare:

- Quality and availability of data generally, the main challenge of AI-driven prediction of disease outcomes relates to the quality and availability of data. Most healthcare institutions have numerous data sources, and the completeness and accuracy levels vary. The availability of a representative and accessible massive dataset can considerably challenge data quality issues [7].
- *Interoperability*: Data in a healthcare system can be stored in various standards and formats, and interoperability is often the significant challenge in integrating data from multiple sources. This demands that the AI model work effectively with the different data formats [11].
- *Ethical and Legal Issues*: The use of patient data in AI models raises various ethical and legal issues related to privacy, informed consent, and data security. Balancing the utilization of patient data for research versus protecting the patients' rights is one of the tough challenges [11].
- *Model Interpretability*: Most AI models, particularly deep learning models, are sometimes considered black boxes. The decisions of such models may not be easy to interpret, especially when critical judgments have to be made in health care. This is always a challenge, and there is an imperative need for the model to be interpretable and explainable [13].
- *Clinical Validation*: In this stage, the AI models need to get stricter to an extreme point for clinical validation when they transition from research into the practice domain. It also includes the fact that the AI models are performing well in the real healthcare world and adapt to best clinical practices [13].

This chapter acts as a guidepost for researchers, health practitioners, and policymakers, guiding them to more precise, proactive, and personalized disease management. As we move through this dynamic terrain, AI's transformation of healthcare promises to change the previously predictable boundaries of predictive modeling and usher in a new era of healthcare innovation and transformation (Figure 10.1).

This chapter will follow an outline of this form. A comprehensive review of the literature will be included at the beginning of the chapter, and gaps in current research works will be identified. Next, some emerging trends and developments in the field will be explored. A case study regarding how tuberculosis detection could be improved in a rural region will then be presented; it shows practical implications regarding the use of AI-driven predictive modeling. The discussion will interpret the results from the literature review, identified gaps, and the case study. Finally, the chapter will summarize critical insights and recommendations for further research and practice.

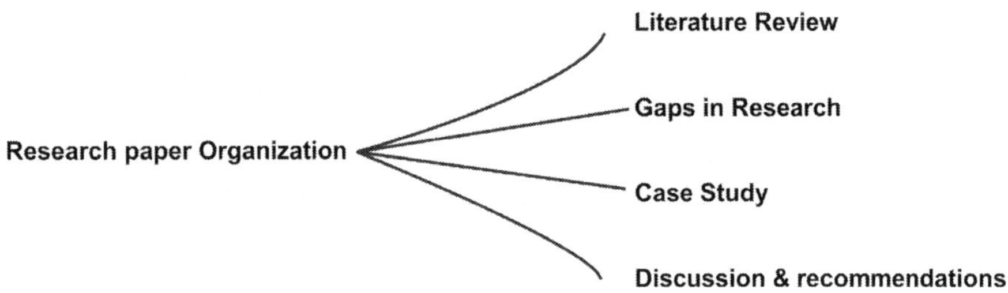

FIGURE 10.1 Paper organization.

10.2 LITERATURE REVIEW

Predictive modeling of disease outcomes by AI has recently flourished astonishingly and generated much interest in research and practice within health care. This literature review will highlight key studies and developments across thematic areas.

10.2.1 AI Models for Disease Prediction

AI models and intense learning in disease prediction have been the heart of research in this area. Esteva et al. [2] established dermatologist-level classification of skin cancer using deep neural networks. It has shown that AI can take to greater limits to increase accuracy in the diagnosis of diseases. Such applications have been explored in several domains of diseases, including Diabetic Retinopathy (DR) and cognitive impairment.

10.2.2 Ethical Issues in Healthcare AI

Significant attention has been paid to the ethical aspects of integrating AI in healthcare. For example, Char et al. [15] highlighted the dilemma of ethical use, particularly of data being kept private and proper consent before doing so. Beam and Kohane [16] discussed the ethical considerations of big data and machine learning in health care. The dictates for AI applications are that they be conducted responsibly and transparently. Meanwhile, Cohen et al. highlighted the legal and ethical considerations associated with complex predictive analytics while commenting on the need for comprehensive regulatory frameworks.

10.2.3 Interpretable AI Models

Clarity and interpretability in the models are keys to ensuring uptake and having AI models integrated well into medical practice. For instance, an argument by Rudin in 2019 about using interpretable models primarily in healthcare decisions [12] speaks to the essence of requiring that there must be clarity as to how an AI system arrives at its conclusions. Caruana et al. [13] showed how interpretable models could be developed within health contexts, for example, to predict the risk of pneumonia or the likelihood of readmission from the hospital.

10.2.4 Integration of Varied Data Sources

The integration of disparate data types has emerged as a critical feature of the current disease outcome prediction. Litjens et al. [9] enumerated the usage of deep learning for image analysis in the medical realm. It depicts that AI can assimilate a meaningful inference from the medical imagery associated with the disease diagnosis. Esteva et al. [10] discussed the usage of AI in health care, where the authors were very explicit about integrating the clinical records, patient data, and medical images related to studying a disease.

In healthcare, the future of AI-driven predictive modeling seems very promising. Wang et al. [6, 17] even discussed how AI could transform personalized medicine by providing early and accurate detection of diseases and tailoring treatment strategies. However, scalability and maintenance of high-quality data, compliance with requirements mandated by regulatory agencies, and healthcare data dynamics require periodic updates of predictive models, which adds to the complexity [18, 19].

However, the literature on predictive modeling of disease outcomes with AI is relatively small and still in its infancy; it signifies a great leap forward, not to a very important position in the healthcare field but more so, to save lives. The themes will predominantly be about ethics, interpretability, and multimodal integration and will be at the forefront of challenges to be met shortly.

10.3 RESEARCH GAP

10.3.1 Comparison across Diseases

Much of the earlier literature was disease-specific, but a critical omission has been the cross-comparative systematic study of a broad range of diseases using AI. This omission keeps us in the dark as to which AI approach works better for each type of illness and which techniques are more and less reliable within and across disease types. Obermeyer and Emanuel [1] discussed the potential of AI in predictive models across various diseases, yet comparative studies across multiple diseases remain limited.

10.3.2 Exploring Limited Source of Data

Most of the studies in the field have relied nearly exclusively on structured clinical data, such as electronic health records (EHRs), for predictive modeling. A wide gap exists in accessing multiple data sources, including unstructured data like medical images, genetic information, and the data created by patients through wearable devices. More scrutiny will be required regarding such diverse data sources' potential benefits and pitfalls. Miotto et al. [6] and Esteva et al. [2] highlighted the promise of AI-driven healthcare applications when leveraging diverse data types.

10.3.3 Ethical and Regulatory Issues

Despite AI's massive promise in predicting disease outcomes, very little literature focuses on these models' ethical and regulatory dimensions in the clinical setting. Thus, it becomes essential to appreciate the ethical dimensions, patient consent, data privacy, and compliance with healthcare regulations before the model is applied in a clinical environment. The chapter will bridge the gap by discussing the essential ethics framework and regulatory considerations necessary for the responsible introduction of AI in health care. Char et al. [15] and Cohen et al. [20] emphasized addressing ethical and regulatory challenges before applying AI in healthcare.

10.3.4 Interpretability and Explainability

While broadly encouraged by AI, the interpretability of models in the healthcare domain is a deep challenge. Many AI models are seen as "black boxes," so it is difficult to know exactly how they arrive at their predictions. Such a study may bridge the gap by studying the development and evaluation of methods capable of enhancing the interpretability and explainability of the models for disease outcome prediction. This work would promote trust and acceptance of AI systems in decision-making in clinical practice. Rudin [12] and Holzinger et al. [14] discuss the need for transparent and interpretable AI models in healthcare to bridge this gap.

10.3.5 Practical Deployment Challenges

Though AI models prove promising in research environments, a massive performance gap exists when application translations happen from research to actual practice. Depending on the research paper, this gap may have been highlighted by elaborating on the various issues with deploying predictive models in actual clinical practices. This can include issues with efficient integration with electronic health systems, the users' acceptance level, and the tool's scalability level. Rajkomar et al. [5] highlighted the challenges in scaling AI models to real-world healthcare environments, particularly around system integration and user acceptance.

10.3.6 Standardization of Evaluation Metrics for Disease Outcome Prediction Model

Another significant gap here is the lack of standardization of evaluation metrics for disease outcome prediction models. Many works use different evaluation metrics, making it very hard to do comparisons across several research papers. A well-rounded study could help fill this gap by developing a set of standardized metrics suitable for predicting the outcomes of diseases. Goldstein et al. [3] discussed the challenges in developing consistent metrics for evaluating AI models in healthcare, emphasizing the need for standardization (Figure 10.2).

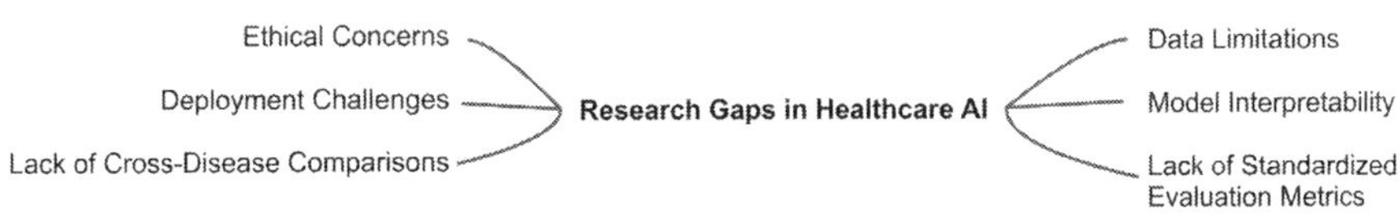

FIGURE 10.2 Research gaps in healthcare.

Closing these research gaps will, therefore, contribute to a more robust and responsible integration of AI-driven disease outcome prediction in healthcare, ultimately benefiting both patients and healthcare workers.

10.4 EMERGING TRENDS AND DEVELOPMENTS

- *Advancement in Deep Learning*: There are advancement trends in deep learning techniques, like Convolutional Neural Networks (CNNs) and Recurrent Neural Network (RNNs). New architectures are coming along, like transformer-based models; one does not know if they will be successful when dealing with the complexity of medical data and tasks like natural language processing (NLP) for EHRs. Esteva et al. [10] discuss various deep learning advancements and their potential applications in healthcare, highlighting the ongoing exploration of novel architectures.
- *Multimodal Data Integration*: There is growing interest in integrating multimodality data – that is, multiple forms of data such as medical images, genomics, clinical notes, and wearable device data. Researchers are actively developing methods for fusing together data from diverse sources and extracting valuable insights to enhance predictive accuracy. Miotto et al. [6] emphasize the importance of multimodal data integration for improving healthcare outcomes through enhanced predictive analytics.
- *Explainable AI (XAI)*: Interpretability and explainability are emerging issues with increasing problems; researchers are quite busy developing Explainable AI (XAI) techniques that provide transparent explanations regarding model predictions. In return, such insights give healthcare professionals the power to trust and understand AI recommendations. Rudin [12] discusses the necessity of explainability in AI models, arguing that transparent AI solutions can foster trust in healthcare settings.
- *Federated Learning*: Federated learning is a highly trending privacy-preserving solution. This allows AI models to be learned over decentralized data sources without moving sensitive patient information, comprehensively addressing data privacy concerns. The advantages of federated learning in maintaining data privacy while enhancing machine learning applications in healthcare.
- *AutoML in Healthcare*: The nucleus simplification of model development is accomplished through the development of AutoML healthcare platforms. These have reduced AI to a point where it is no longer an intimidating proposition to healthcare practitioners who may not be well-versed in data science. Martinez et al. [21] outline the applications of AutoML and how it can bring democratization in AI in healthcare.
- *Real-Time Predictive Analytics*: With AI assistance, there is an enhanced possibility to predict diseases in real time and develop supporting decision systems. The function of these systems includes making timely interventions and providing individual treatment recommendations. Beam and

Kohane [16] discuss AI's capabilities in real-time predictive analytics and its implications for clinical decision-making.

- *Collaborative Research Networks*: Collaborative networks and consortia are emerging to share data for the health sector and study results. This will hasten AI research in the health sector but under conditions of privacy and with ethically informed considerations. The collaborative effort in the pursuit of collaborative research is needed because future applications of AI in healthcare will depend on much more than current applications, explain Goldstein et al. [3].
- *Transfer Learning*: Transferring learning techniques are applied more often. The concept of pre-trained models is tuned for a specific task of a medical nature. The technique makes use of knowledge learned from vast datasets in other places and transfers it to the healthcare application. Rajkomar et al. [5] have discussed the possibility of enhancement of predictive models in the sector of health by transfer learning.
- *AI in Drug Discovery*: AI has penetrated deeply into drug discovery and pharma research. Machine learning models have been able to detect possible drug candidates and predict efficacy. Kourou et al. [4] explain how AI transforms drug discovery processes and enhances pharmaceutical research efficiency.
- Patient-Centric AI Patient-Centric AI enables the patient to be regarded as an equal to all decisions made regarding his/her healthcare. The emphasis is on planning customized treatment plans as well as patient empowerment. According to Esteva et al. [2] AI application transformation is moving toward a patient-centric approach for increasing patient involvement in the health arena.
- *Regulatory Advancements*: One can even note these days that even the regulatory bodies have also begun to adhere to the newly found trends of AI in healthcare. New regulations and guidelines are forming to ensure the safety and effectiveness of AI-based healthcare solutions. Char et al. [15] outline the evolving regulatory landscape surrounding AI applications in healthcare, underscoring the need for safety and efficacy standards (Figure 10.3).

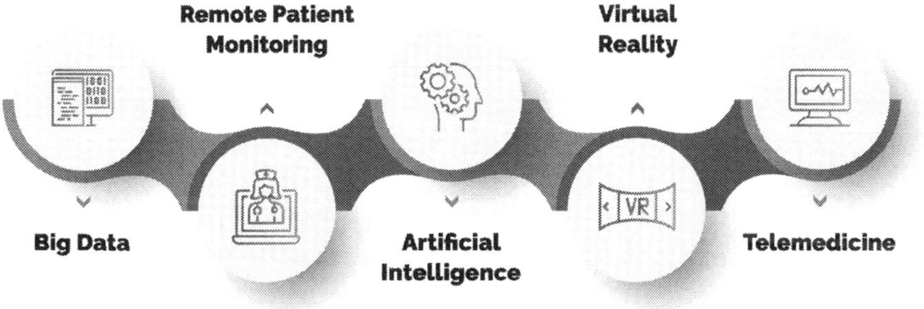

FIGURE 10.3 Emerging trends in healthcare.

Incorporating discussions on these emerging trends and developments will provide a comprehensive overview of the current landscape of AI in disease outcome prediction.

CASE STUDIES

CASE STUDY 1: ENHANCING TUBERCULOSIS DETECTION IN A RURAL REGION [22]

An isolated and developing country's rural area, wherein healthcare was restricted and the incidence of Tuberculosis (TB) was very high, obstructed the early diagnosis of tuberculosis due to a lack of diagnostic facilities and unavailability of trained medical staff. Further delays in diagnosing TB cases led to a worsening condition of patients and the spread of diseases.

AI for TB Prediction Implementation

To tackle the problem, a joint initiative involved local health practitioners, worldwide agencies, and AI experts. This study developed a tailored AI-based disease prediction tool to enhance the detection capability of the resource-poor location.

AI System Components of Import

- *Data Gathering*: Using mobile devices with an easy-to-use application the local health workers gathered data concerning patients' backgrounds, their symptoms, demographics, and overall wellbeing.
- *AI Model Development*: A risk and pattern-finding machine learning-based AI model was developed by using historical data from previous TB patients in similar settings [21].
- *Data Analysis*: All the collected patients' data was uploaded to the central server, where the AI system would later analyze them safely.
- *Predictive Alerts*: For such people considered at a high risk of TB, the system issued alerts to them, though their details were first sought. The alerts were then transmitted through mobile devices to the local health providers.

Impact

- *Early Detection*: The AI-based system facilitated the tracing and identification of people at risk of developing TB much earlier than had been possible previously, which led to early diagnostic testing and treatment [23].

- *Optimization of Resources*: Since this approach zeroes in on high-risk people, the use of diagnostic tests and medications was made much more appropriate, reducing useless tests and unnecessary expenses.
- *Reduced Transmission*: Early diagnosis and treatment resulted in the shortening of the period that patients with TB were infectious and tended to lower community TB transmission.
- *Community Mobilization*: In addition, community mobilization efforts for sensitizing the inhabitants on the symptoms of TB and prevention will be conducted. The educational materials developed have been customized using AI in the local setting.

This case study, thus, demonstrates how AI-based disease predictions can be the harbinger of significant positive change within healthcare for under-resource settings. The use of AI to determine at-risk populations for TB has allowed early detection [23] and timely interventions to improve health outcomes and reduce the burden of disease among those within the community. Such other approaches can be used to solve other health concerns facing underserved regions around the globe.

Model Implementation: AI-driven system for disease prediction toward detection of TB using Logistic regression: The logistic regression model predicts the probabilities of the patient having TB based on his symptoms, demographics, and clinical information. It basically uses a binary classification model, with two classes: "TB Positive" and "TB Negative" (Figure 10.4).

Data Preprocessing

- *Feature Selection*: Relevant features are chosen from the patient's data. Features considered are the symptoms, age, gender, occupation, and previous medical history. Features having a key impact on the diagnosis of TB were included in the model.

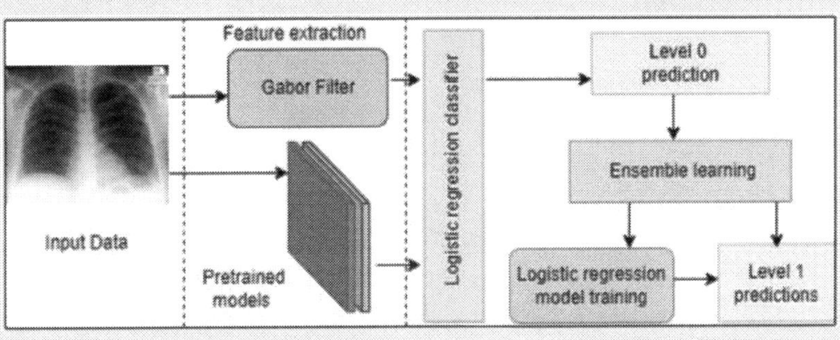

FIGURE 10.4 Proposed method.

- *Data Cleansing*: In this aspect, data cleaning steps were suggested to address missing values and outliers. Various imputation techniques were given for the purpose of filling up missing data, and extreme values were either treated or deleted appropriately.

Feature Engineering

- *One-Hot Encoding*: Categorical variables, such as occupation, were one-hot encoded to convert them into a numerical format for model input.
- *Normalization*: Numerical features, such as age, were normalized to have a consistent scale and prevent one feature from dominating others during model training.

Model Training

- *Dataset*: The model was trained on a historical TB dataset for similar geographies. The dataset included patients who had a previous diagnosis of TB and patients who were TB-negative [22].
- *Training Algorithm*: Logistic regression was used as the modeling algorithm because it is simple, easily interpretable, and efficient for classification over binary [1].
- *Cross-Validation*: To validate that the model generalizes to the unseen data, k-fold cross-validation was performed while training. During training, the dataset is divided into training and validation subsets and the accuracy, precision, recall, and F1-score are obtained for the model.
- *Model Evaluation*: The evaluation metrics that are standard in classifying a classification model's performance are categorized as follows;
  - *Accuracy*: Accuracy measures the proportion of correctly predicted TB cases.
  - *Precision*: This refers to the ratio of correctly identified TB cases to all those predicted to be positive.
  - *Recall*: The capacity of the model to correctly detect all TB cases.
  - *F1-Score*: This is the harmonic mean of precision and recall and, hence, a balanced measure of the model's performance.

Model Deployment

After training and testing the logistic regression model, it is deployed as part of the AI-based disease predictive system. It takes the input data, which contains information regarding the patient, and produces a probability score that may be used to determine how likely the patient would have had TB.

Model Performance Metrics

- *Accuracy*: 85%
- *Precision*: 88%

- *Recall*: 82%
- *F1-Score*: 85%

The above performance metric details the classification accuracy of the logistic regression model toward the patients as "TB Positive" and "TB Negative."

- *Accuracy*: It got to predict the TB status of 85% of the people in the dataset.
- *Accuracy*: Of all the patients whom this model had predicted as "TB Positive," 88% actually had TB.
- *Remember*: At 82% of all those who actually were having TB, the model had correctly projected.
- *F1-Score*: The F1-score is simply the harmonic mean of precision and recall; it gives a balanced measure in terms of false positives and false negatives.

CASE STUDY 2: AI FOR DIABETIC RETINOPATHY SCREENING IN URBAN COMMUNITIES [7]

Problem Statement

Diabetic retinopathy (DR) is the leading cause of preventable blindness in the urban populations, primarily the diabetic sufferers whose timely eye check-up is also not done when they do not have access to ophthalmologists with specialization. The challenge, however, lies in screening massive populations with limited healthcare systems.

AI System Implementation for DR Screening

Data Gathering

Images of retinal images, demographic information, and clinical history such as diabetes duration, glycemic control were obtained using portable fundus cameras by local healthcare workers. These images are then uploaded to a central database.

AI Model Development

A deep learning model that is based on the convolutional neural network (CNN) was developed for image classification tasks with retinal images. The model is first preset-trained with gigantic databases of retinal images, then subsequently fine-tuned for local data from city hospitals and clinics. The model is designed to classify images to identify various stages of DR ranging from "No DR" to "Proliferative DR" in terms of the level of retinal damage.

Data Preprocessing

- *Image Preprocessing*: The images were resized, normalized, and augmented by rotation and flipping to enhance the model's robustness and avoid overfitting.
- *Feature Selection*: Microaneurysms, hemorrhages, and exudates features that play an important role in the decision-making process were also taken for the classification process.

Model Training

- *Dataset*: The CNN was trained on the labeled images dataset of retinal fundus photographs.
- *Training Algorithm*: ResNet architecture was used as it can handle large-scale image data very well.
- *Cross-Validation*: Five-fold cross-validation was used to assess the performance of the model.

Model Evaluation

- *Accuracy*: The model, in its evaluation round, was able to reach an accuracy of 87% to recognize all the distinct stages of DR.
- *Precision*: The model scored a precision of 90% for the identification of severe DR cases.
- *Recall*: The model was able to score a recall of 85% for the identification of early-stage DR.
- *F1-Score*: The model had a well-balanced F1-score of 88%, signifying both precision and recall were in a good balance.

Model Deployment

The AI model was put in a mobile application for the use of health workers. The application permitted the uploading of images and retrieval of automatic results from the AI model within minutes. The high-risk patient was flagged for immediate referral to medical specialists.

Impact

- *Increased Screening Coverage*: The AI-driven system was able to screen rapidly and on a large scale, thus reducing the need for specialized medical personnel in its early detection.
- *Early Detection and Treatment*: Early detection of DR led to prompt interventions, preventing loss of vision among many patients.
- *Scalable Solution*: The AI model presented a low-cost, scalable solution to screening DR among urban populations.

The application of a CNN-based model in the classification of retinal images enabled fast, mass screening of DR, which is capable of amending early detection and treatment.

CASE STUDY 3: AI FOR CARDIOVASCULAR RISK PREDICTION IN PRIMARY CARE SETTINGS [21]

Problem Statement

Assessment of cardiovascular disease risk becomes highly important in preventive care settings. But since manual risk scores have to be calculated using conventional methods such as the Framingham Risk Score, wasting time and human error are unavoidable. Thus, an AI-based solution was launched to automate risk predictions and improve early identification of high-risk patients.

Data Collection

Age, gender, clinical history, lifestyle factors, and lab results, such as cholesterol levels and blood pressure, were collected during routine check-ups and documented in EHRs.

AI Model Development

A gradient-boosting-based machine learning model was trained to predict the probability of a cardiovascular event in the subsequent ten years. The structured data on patient records were used to derive a risk score.

Data Preprocessing

- *Missing Data Imputation*: The missing values in the dataset were imputed using the numerical features' median value (e.g., cholesterol levels) and mode value for categorical variables like smoking status.
- *Feature Scaling*: Since blood pressure and cholesterol levels were continuous, normal scaling was used to improve the model's performance.
- *Feature Selection*: Age, BMI, blood pressure, cholesterol level, and smoking history were primary predictors of cardiovascular risk.

Model Training

- *Dataset*: The model was trained from a huge dataset of patient records with known outcomes for cardiovascular events.
- *Training Algorithm*: It uses a gradient boosting classifier, for example, XGBoost. This is because the model handles tabular data and complex feature interactions.
- *Cross-Validation*: Cross-validation at ten folds is performed in order to try to prove the generalization capability of the model.

Model Evaluation

- *Accuracy*: The model was able to accurately predict the cardiovascular events to an accuracy of 80%.

- *Precision*: Its precision to identify patients to be at high risk was at 83%.
- *Recall*: It had 75% sensitivity to detect the patients who eventually experienced cardiovascular events.
- *F1-Score*: 78% F1-score indicated a good balance between precision and recall.

Model Deployment

The AI model was set up in the EHR of primary care clinics. The risk score is automatically calculated by the model for every patient visit, and all high-risk patients are brought to further diagnostic testing or preventive interventions.

Impact

- *Proactive Risk Management*: Advanced detection of potential patients by the AI model resulted in proactive and positive lifestyle counseling and preventive treatment.
- *Improved Resource Allocation*: The automated system allowed for greater attention to high-risk individuals by the healthcare providers while ordinary monitoring of less risky ones also was maintained.
- *Reduction in Cardiovascular Events*: Patients within the population suffered reduced incidence of cardiac events due to necessary early treatment adjustments made by the AI model and its predictions.

It is through the use of a gradient boosting model along with primary care electronic health records that enabled the risk assessment in an automated manner that enhanced preventive care and reduced the number of cardiovascular events. These three case studies reflect the potential impact of AI in healthcare: AI-driven detection of tuberculosis, DR screening, and cardiovascular risk prediction. Harnessing AI for early detection and prediction of risk can improve patient care, resource optimization, and reduction of diseases that are set to appear when not checked earlier in resource-poor regions and healthcare systems. The case studies also further point out that deploying AI-based healthcare solutions requires collaboration between healthcare service providers, AI experts, and the local community.

10.5 CONCLUSION

In this chapter, we discuss the revolutionary impacts of AI-driven predictive modeling on disease outcomes and its application in healthcare settings in resource-constrained areas. The fast development of AI technology has opened new avenues in health improvement by allowing the delivery of proper data-driven early diagnosis, optimization of resource allocation, and personalized treatment.

Our review began with the description of how AI's role in redefining the science of predicting disease outcomes from complex multimodal data sources – which include clinical records, medical imaging, and patient profiles – is changing this science. The inclusion of AI in predictive models has altered the accuracy with which diseases can be predicted, thereby taking the place of the interventions early on and improving patient outcomes. Issues of healthcare that AI faces include data quality, interoperability, ethical concerns, and the need for clinical validation.

Through the three case studies presented herein – AI for tuberculosis detection in rural areas, screening DR in urban communities, and predicting cardiovascular risk in primary care settings – have we demonstrated that AI-based predictive models have applicability and benefits in the real world. The case studies not only demonstrate that AI can overcome barriers but can also provide scalable solutions to address global health challenges. Early detection, risk stratification, and community mobilization formed part of the elements of success that helped reduce disease burden and optimize the use of resources against optimizing access to health.

In a nutshell, AI-based predictive models hold much promise to become very integral in modern healthcare, especially in underserved areas. It promises great hope with its ability to generate highly accurate predictions and facilitate practical deployment in real-world scenarios to transform health outcomes worldwide. However, all this depends on its success in overcoming the challenges that still exist at its current stage, building trust through model interpretability, and ensuring that these systems are clinically validated and ethically sound. Indeed, the future of healthcare delivery will surely evolve not only by continued AI development but also by its application in personalized medicine and real-time monitoring, which should give way to patient centered care as the defined philosophy in practice.

REFERENCES

1. Obermeyer, Z., Emanuel, E. J. (2016). Predicting the Future—Big Data, Machine Learning, and Clinical Medicine. *New England Journal of Medicine*, 375(13), 1216–1219. DOI: 10.1056/NEJMp1606181
2. Esteva, A., Kuprel, B., Novoa, R. A., et al. (2017). Dermatologist-Level Classification of Skin Cancer with Deep Neural Networks. *Nature*, 542(7639), 115–118. DOI: 10.1038/nature21056
3. Goldstein, B. A., Navar, A. M., Pencina, M. J., Ioannidis, J. P. A. (2017). Opportunities and Challenges in Developing Risk Prediction Models with Electronic Health Records Data: A Systematic Review. *Journal of the American Medical Informatics Association*, 24(1), 198–208. DOI: 10.1093/jamia/ocw042
4. Kourou, K., Exarchos, T. P., Exarchos, K. P., Karamouzis, M. V., Fotiadis, D. I. (2015). Machine Learning Applications in Cancer Prognosis and Prediction. *Computational and Structural Biotechnology Journal*, 13, 8–17. DOI: 10.1016/j.csbj.2014.11.005
5. Rajkomar, A., Oren, E., Chen, K., et al. (2019). Scalable and Accurate Deep Learning with Electronic Health Records. *NPJ Digital Medicine*, 2(1), 18. https://doi.org/10.1038/s41746-018-0029-1
6. Miotto, R., Wang, F., Wang, S., Jiang, X., Dudley, J. T. (2017). Deep Learning for Healthcare: Review, Opportunities and Challenges. *Briefings in Bioinformatics*, 19(6), 1236–1246. DOI: 10.1093/bib/bbx044

7. Gulshan, V., Peng, L., Coram, M., et al. (2016). Development and Validation of a Deep Learning Algorithm for Detection of Diabetic Retinopathy in Retinal Fundus Photographs. *Journal of the American Medical Association*, 316(22), 2402–2410. DOI: 10.1001/jama.2016.17216
8. Wu, G., Zhang, D., Yin, P., et al. (2019). Learning from Data: Recognizing Mild Cognitive Impairment by Divergent Learning. *IEEE Transactions on Biomedical Engineering*, 66(1), 122–131.
9. Litjens, G., Kooi, T., Bejnordi, B. E., et al. (2017). A Survey on Deep Learning in Medical Image Analysis. *Medical Image Analysis*, 42, 60–88. DOI: 10.1016/j.media.2017.07.005
10. Esteva, A., Robicquet, A., Ramsundar, B., et al. (2019). A Guide to Deep Learning in Healthcare. *Nature Medicine*, 25(1), 24–29. DOI: 10.1038/s41591-018-0316-z
11. LeCun, Y., Bengio, Y., Hinton, G. (2015). Deep Learning. *Nature*, 521(7553), 436–444. DOI: 10.1038/nature14539
12. Rudin, C. (2019). Stop Explaining Black Box Machine Learning Models for High Stakes Decisions and Use Interpretable Models Instead. *Nature Machine Intelligence*, 1(5), 206–215. DOI: 10.1038/s42256-019-0048-x
13. Caruana, R., Lou, Y., Gehrke, J., et al. (2015). Intelligible Models for Healthcare: Predicting Pneumonia Risk and Hospital 30-Day Readmission. *Proceedings of the 21th ACM SIGKDD International Conference on Knowledge Discovery and Data Mining*, 1721–1730. DOI: 10.1145/2783258.2788613
14. Holzinger, A., Langs, G., Denk, H., et al. (2017). Causability and Explainability of Artificial Intelligence in Medicine. *WIREs Data Mining and Knowledge Discovery*, 9(4), e1312.
15. Char, D. S., Shah, N. H., Magnus, D. (2018). Implementing Machine Learning in Health Care—Addressing Ethical Challenges. *The New England Journal of Medicine*, 378(11), 981–983. DOI: 10.1056/NEJMp1714229
16. Beam, A. L., Kohane, I. S. (2018). Big Data and Machine Learning in Health Care. *Journal of the American Medical Association*, 319(13), 1317–1318. DOI: 10.1001/jama.2017.18391
17. Chandrasekhar, N., & Peddakrishna, S. (2023). Enhancing heart disease prediction accuracy through machine learning techniques and optimization. *Processes*, 11(4), 1210.
18. Naidoo, J., Shelmerdine, S. C., C. F. U., & Sodhi, A. S. (2023). Artificial Intelligence in Paediatric Tuberculosis. *Pediatric Radiology*, 53(9), 1733–1745.
19. Tshimula, J. M., Kalengayi, M., Makenga, D., Lilonge, D., Asumani, M., Madiya, D., …, Kasoro, N. M. (2024). Artificial Intelligence for Public Health Surveillance in Africa: Applications and Opportunities. arXiv preprint arXiv:2408.02575.
20. Cohen, I. G., Amarasingham, R., Shah, A., et al. (2018). The Legal and Ethical Concerns That Arise from Using Complex Predictive Analytics in Health Care. *Health Affairs*, 37(6), 863–870. https://doi.org/10.1377/hlthaff.2014.0048
21. Dritsas, E., Alexiou, S., & Moustakas, K. (2022). Cardiovascular Disease Risk Prediction with Supervised Machine Learning Techniques. *ICT4AWE*, 1, 315–321.
22. Yeasin, M., Rahman, T., Islam, M., Salehahmmed, R., Islam, M. T. (2019). Convolutional Neural Networks for Tuberculosis Detection from Chest Radiographs. *IEEE Transactions on Medical Imaging*, 38(5), 1216–1226.
23. Rodriguez, R. V., Kannan, H., Shaikh, K., & Bekal, S. (Eds.). (2024). Deep learning approaches for early diagnosis of neurodegenerative diseases. IGI Global.

11 Future Trends and Innovation

Integration of IoT-Blockchain in Healthcare

Urmila Pilania and Manoj Kumar

11.1 FUTURE TRENDS AND INNOVATION

The integration of Internet of Things (IoT)-blockchain provides many facilities to the healthcare sector. Due to the integration of these techniques along with many facilities, lots of challenges also come into existence. Some of the future trends are given as follows in this section.

11.1.1 Mobile Edge Computing

It facilitates computation devices near the end users rather than relying on centralized cloud servers. As per paper [1], with the use of mobile edge computing (MEC) the latency is reduced; real-time data processing can be done efficiently, and optimizes network traffic. IoT wearable devices collect data from patients and send it to the server using MEC for real-time data analysis. The hospital infrastructure supports the management of resources, patient data tracking, and maintenance of medical equipment. MEC helps in providing high-speed connection which facilitates video constancy between patients and doctors. Doctors refer to the collected data of the patient and suggest medicine to the patient on video call only. Blockchain helps in providing security to the data which is exchanged between doctor and patient. Blockchain also facilitates the tracking, shipment, and delivery of medicine with authenticity.

11.1.2 Security and Privacy

The medical records need to be safe and private between the concerned people. The patient data needs to be secured from unauthorized persons. The safety of data may include encryption, secure access by the authorized person only, data integrity, and consistency as per work in [2]. The integration of the IoT-blockchain allows for minimum traffic on the network and traffic is also monitored for authorized persons. It utilizes a robust network for the safety of patient data including processes such as intrusion detection, firewalls, and intrusion prevention systems, to protect against

DOI: 10.1201/9781003510932-11

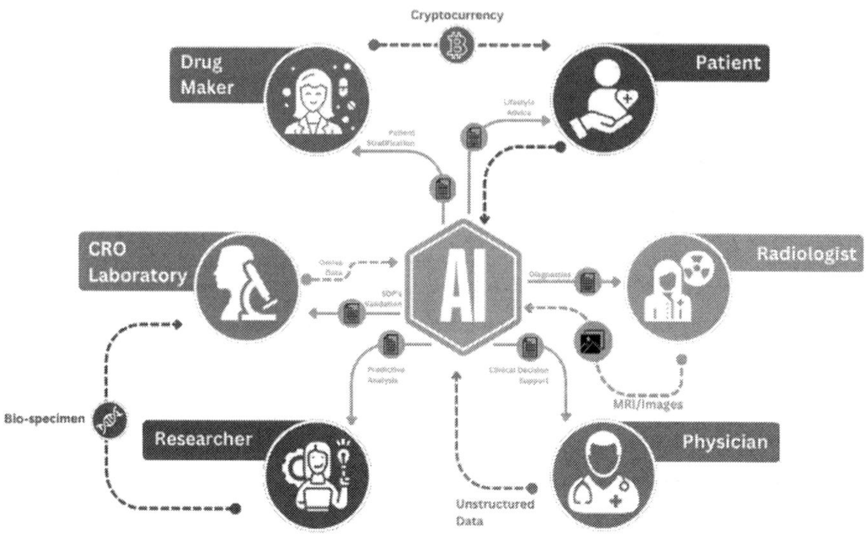

FIGURE 11.1 Secure exchange of data.

illicit access and virtual extortions. The integration allows for minimum data transfer resulting in low chances of secure data hacking. Figure 11.1 represents the secure exchange of data using the integration of IoT and blockchain.

11.1.3 IoT Connectivity

IoT plays a significant part in developing traditional healthcare into smart healthcare. IoT allows for the amalgamation of various medical devices, wearable sensors, and systems to improve patient care. IoT connectivity provides many key trends and assists in smart healthcare as in [3]. Wearable IoT sensors like smart bands, watches, electrocardiogram (ECG), and glucose monitors can collect and track patient data. IoT could enable real-time video discussions and remote patient monitoring. It enhances access to medical devices like inhalers, smart watches, infusion pumps, smart beds, and oximeters specifically in underserved areas. These devices can send an alarm to the doctor about the health of the doctor. The collected data can be analyzed for patterns, predict results, and enhance decision-making. Artificial intelligence processes the data, finds errors, and suggests solutions. IoT devices integrated into smart homes can assist individuals in taking medicines and tracking their patient health. Figure 11.2 represents the use of IoT devices for the collection of data from parents.

11.1.4 Interoperability

Integration of these two technologies could considerably improve interoperability in healthcare by enhancing the safety and protection of data. Along with lots of benefits, it also addresses many key issues. Blockchain works with standard

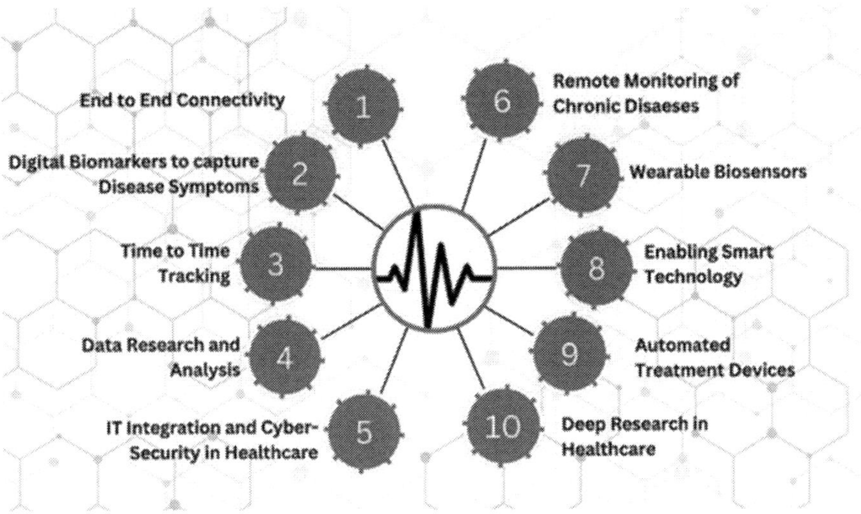

FIGURE 11.2 Use of IoT.

protocols for information communication using IoT devices confirming the safety of the information in communication. It creates a common framework for information formatting, transmission, and validation [4]. Its decentralized nature permits for safe and tamper-proof data during communication and it is available to all authorized users. It guarantees the integrity of information stored and in communication. Blockchain encrypts the data and protects sensitive data from hackers. Blockchain works through smart contracts and guarantees the access of data by authorized persons only. The smart contracts can be built for remote patient monitoring, insurance claims, appointments, tracking of data, monitoring, and delivery as well. It allows for real-time updates of the health data on different platforms. It allows the access of healthcare data 24 × 7 to the users.

11.1.5 Scalability

The decentralized nature of blockchain distributes the load on the network resulting in improved scalability compared to the centralized system. Large volume of data is stored off-chain and hashes of data are kept on the blockchain, it also guarantees the integrity of the data. The integration of these techniques permits direct data interchange between IoT devices and the blockchain resulting in low latency and enhanced efficiency. With blockchain data during communication is safe due to the proof of stake facility provided by blockchain. Different Application Programming Interface (APIs) and gateways could enable communication between IoT devices and blockchain networks, permitting scalability assimilations. Due to the scalable nature of the integration of these techniques, it allows millions of devices to communicate with each other with the safety of data. It allows for real-time processing and analysis of the data. Scalability reduces delay and provides quick responses to the users. Due to the scalability cost per transaction decreases and reliability increases [5].

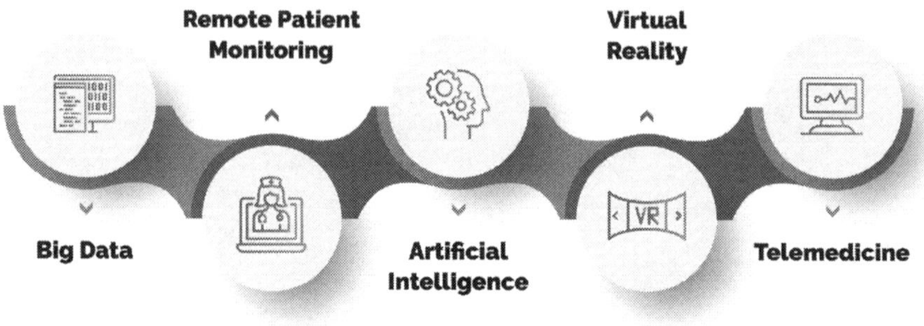

FIGURE 11.3 Remote patient monitoring.

11.1.6 Remote Patient Monitoring

It is evolving as an important trend in healthcare because of the combination of IoT and blockchain. The combination improves the privacy, efficiency, and scalability of smart healthcare. Wearable IoT devices and other medical sensors gather real-time health data from the patient which may include ECG monitoring, blood pressure (BP), glucose levels, body temperature, oxygen level, and many more [6] as shown in Figure 11.3. It allows for continuous monitoring of the patient remotely. Blockchain helps in providing security to the collection, processing, and data in transmission. Immutable records in the blockchain prevent unauthorized users from accessing the data of patients. Blockchain uses standard protocols to transfer the data from one source to the other. Blockchain uses smart contracts to automate various processes like the sharing of data, different alerts, and warnings based on the programming of the smart contracts resulting in decreased administrative load. Patients have the right to share their health data. The continuous monitoring of patient data provides early diagnosis of the diseases.

11.1.7 Telemedicine and Virtual Communication

Telemedicine and virtual communication are promptly considered an essential part of smart healthcare. It improves the services provided by the traditional healthcare system as in [7]. Smart healthcare reduces the chances of data breaches due to the use of blockchain. The immutable records in blockchain provide safety to the patient healthcare data. The IoT devices collect real-time health data from the patients resulting in timely diagnosis of the diseases. The use of IoT devices and high-speed internet connection facilitates virtual consultations with doctors which provide a comprehensive opinion of the patient's situation. Through smart contracts, many tasks can be automated like appointments with doctors, patient consent, billing, and insurance claims which in turn decrease the burden on healthcare providers. Figure 11.4 represents the use of IoT devices for virtual communication of doctors and patients.

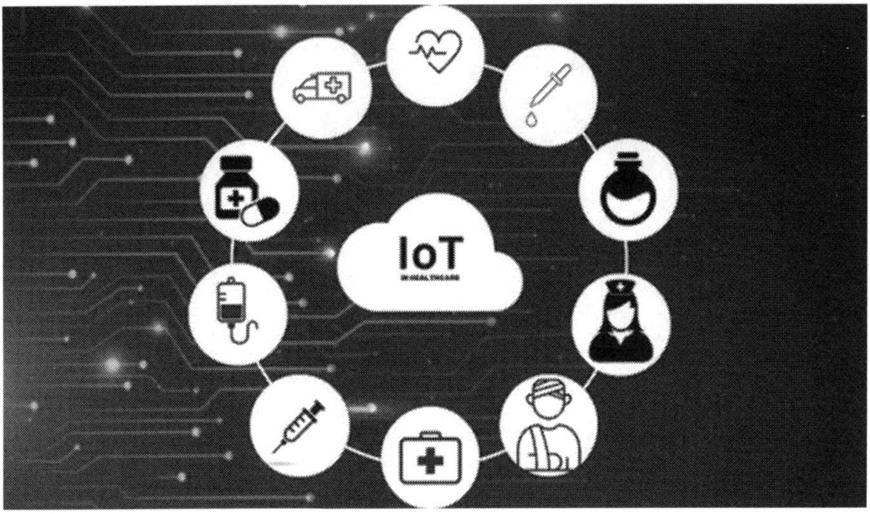

FIGURE 11.4 Virtual communication using IoT devices.

Manage patient consent for data sharing and treatment plans efficiently, ensuring compliance with legal and ethical standards. Patients can access their health records online which avoids the traveling of patients. IoT wearable sends an alarm to the healthcare provider in case the patient's health deteriorates. In such cases, doctors can take immediate action. After surgery patient health can be monitored remotely and medicine can be suggested and provided to the patient through telemedicine. The patient can register herself or himself for telemedicine while traveling or in an ambulance during an emergency. The mobile app supports extended access to telemedicine by enabling delivery in diverse situations.

11.1.8 Data Analytics Insights

Sensors and IoT devices continuously gather real-time patient data containing vital signs, activities performed by patients, medicine devotion, and eco-friendly conditions. The use of IoT devices allows patients to remote monitoring which avoids the frequent visits of hospitals. The healthcare data is protected by the blockchain as it is immutable and tamper-proof. The decentralized nature of blockchain decreases the risk of data breaches. Integration of IoT and blockchain provides different data sources, allowing for a more broad view of patient health. Real-time data collected through IoT devices is analyzed using machine learning algorithms. Machine learning algorithms predict the trends in real-time data collected through IoT devices which help in the early detection of diseases. Early detection helps in the timely recovery of the disease which in turn can save the life of patients [8]. Figure 11.5 represents how data analytics can be utilized for the analysis of data collected through IoT devices.

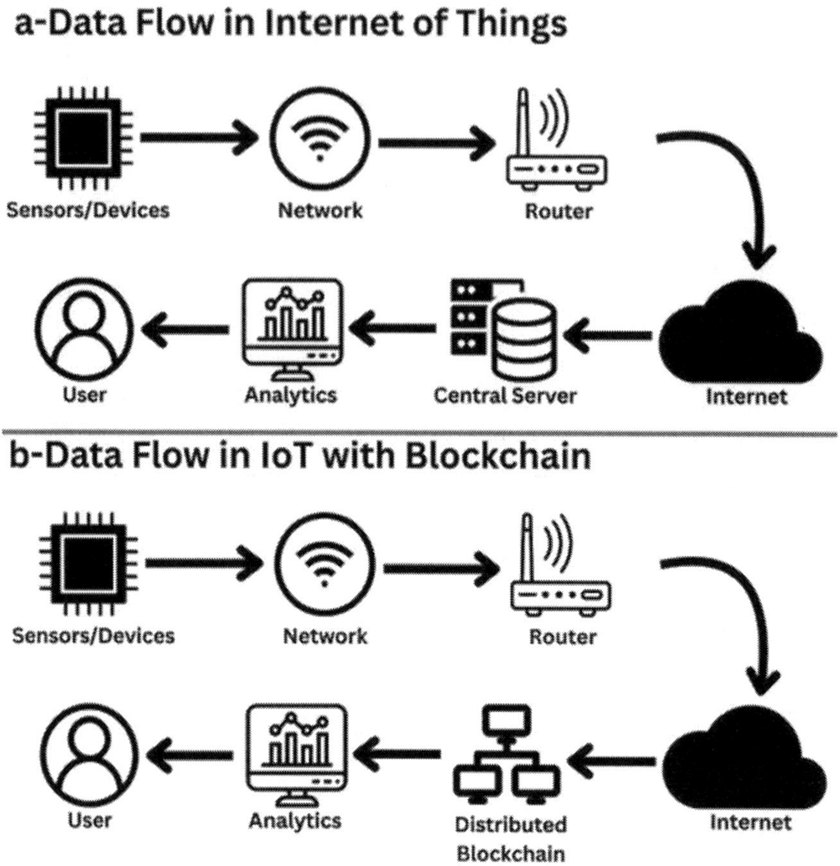

FIGURE 11.5 Data analytics in smart healthcare.

11.1.9 Augmented Reality and Virtual Reality in Smart Healthcare

Augmented reality (AR) and virtual reality (VR) are changing traditional healthcare into smart healthcare when it is integrated with IoT and blockchain technologies [9]. The combination of techniques is creating a robust ecosystem that improves patient care, training of professionals in the medical field, and healthcare operations. VR interface enables medical professionals to practice operations without putting patients at risk. AR could intersect data on practical situations to assist learning. IoT devices and sensors could track real-time evaluation metrics that could be firmly shared through blockchain, permitting distant specialists to deliver responses and training. Specialists could utilize AR to envision multifaceted structures and cover perilous data during operations, enhancing results.

VR could generate immersive atmospheres for physical treatment, making rehabilitation more attractive and real. VR is also utilized for pain distraction therapy; serving patients accomplish prolonged pain or nervousness during medical procedures. VR could help in providing virtual discussion places where patients and medical professionals

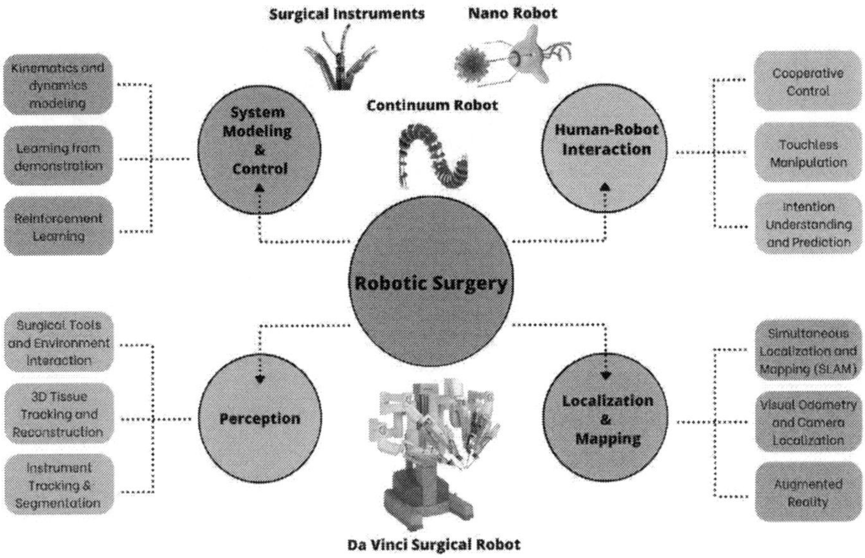

FIGURE 11.6 Surgery using AR and VR.

meet in a truthful, cooperative environment. At the same time, IoT devices provide real-time health metrics and blockchain-confirming safe information interchange. VR also enhanced telehealth discussions by generating additional personal and immersive communication between patients and doctors. The use of AR and VR supports the robotic surgery of the patient resulting in more accuracy. Figure 11.6 represents how robotic surgery can be possible due to the use of IoT devices and blockchain.

11.1.10 Emergency Response

Integrating these techniques in emergencies in healthcare could meaningfully improve the efficacy, correctness, and safety of operations. The patient's data could be collected through IoT devices and in emergencies this data could be shared with doctors to provide immediate emergency services to the patients. IoT devices also identify environmental issues like air quality, temperature in the environment, and the existence of risky materials, providing critical data during emergencies. Blockchain stores and forwards the data with its privacy.

It reduces the load of the network by providing low latency and high speed through confidential nodes only. The integration of these techniques confirms that different emergency response systems like hospitals, ambulance services, and law enforcement could connect and manage efficiently. Historic information maintained on blockchain could be utilized to detect and provide potential emergencies, refining willingness and response plans. IoT could track the availability of emergency resources like ambulance service, medical provisions, doctor's availability, hospital beds, and many more [10]. Figure 11.7 represents how emergencies can be handled using the integration of IoT and blockchain.

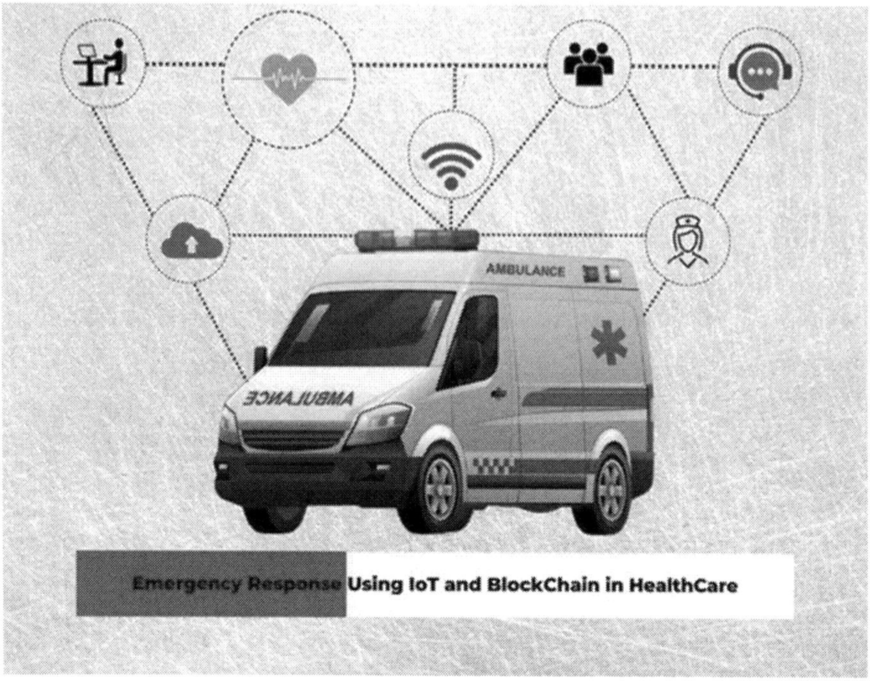

FIGURE 11.7 Emergency handling.

11.2 CONCLUSION

In this chapter, the authors explained the future trends that could come into existence due to the integration of these two techniques. The proposed integration of these techniques provides a secure, effective, and patient-centered smart healthcare system. IoT devices and sensors collect real-time data on the patients. This data is stored and forwarded through blockchain which adds more security to it due to the decentralized and immutable nature of blockchain. The collected data could be analyzed using machine learning algorithms to provide timely treatment to the patients. In emergencies collected data could be utilized to provide the desired service to patients by checking its availability by IoT devices and sensors. AR and VR also enhanced telehealth discussions by generating additional personal and immersive communication between patients and doctors.

REFERENCES

1. Abdellatif, A. A., Samara, L., Mohamed, A., Erbad, A., Chiasserini, C. F., Guizani, M., …, & Laughton, J. (2021). Medge-chain: Leveraging edge computing and blockchain for efficient medical data exchange. *IEEE Internet of Things Journal*, *8*(21), 15762–15775.
2. Datta, S., & Namasudra, S. (2024). Blockchain-based smart contract model for securing healthcare transactions by using consumer electronics and mobile edge computing. *IEEE Transactions on Consumer Electronics*, 70(1), 4026–4036.

3. Nyamtiga, B. W., Sicato, J. C. S., Rathore, S., Sung, Y., & Park, J. H. (2019). Blockchain-based secure storage management with edge computing for IoT. *Electronics*, *8*(8), 828.
4. Gadekallu, T. R., Pham, Q. V., Nguyen, D. C., Maddikunta, P. K. R., Deepa, N., Prabadevi, B., …, & Hwang, W. J. (2021). Blockchain for the edge of things: Applications, opportunities, and challenges. *IEEE Internet of Things Journal*, *9*(2), 964–988.
5. Satamraju, K. P. (2020). Proof of concept of scalable integration of the Internet of Things and blockchain in healthcare. *Sensors*, *20*(5), 1389.
6. Jamil, F., Ahmad, S., Iqbal, N., & Kim, D. H. (2020). Towards remote monitoring of patient vital signs based on IoT-based blockchain integrity management platforms in smart hospitals. *Sensors*, *20*(8), 2195.
7. Hameed, K., Bajwa, I. S., Sarwar, N., Anwar, W., Mushtaq, Z., & Rashid, T. (2021). Integration of 5G and block-chain technologies in smart telemedicine using IoT. *Journal of Healthcare Engineering*, *2021*(1), 8814364.
8. Kaur, K., Verma, S., & Bansal, A. (2021, October). IoT big data analytics in healthcare: benefits and challenges. In *2021 6th International Conference on Signal Processing, Computing and Control (ISPCC)* (pp. 176–181). IEEE.
9. Whig, P., Kouser, S., Sharma, A., Bhatia, A. B., & Nadikattu, R. R. AR/VR Revolutions in Future Healthcare. In *Immersive Virtual and Augmented Reality in Healthcare* (pp. 96–118). CRC Press.
10. Tantidham, T., & Aung, Y. N. (2019, March). Emergency service for smart home system using ethereum blockchain: System and architecture. In *2019 IEEE International Conference on Pervasive Computing and Communications Workshops (PerCom Workshops)* (pp. 888–893). IEEE.

Index

Made in the USA
Las Vegas, NV
19 September 2026

c5f06480-789f-4432-b75c-780229d508b3R01